RENAL DIET COOKBOOK

A Beginner's Guide To Managing Kidney Disease With Low-Sodium, Low-Potassium, And Low-Phosphorous Recipes

HELEN WILLIAMS

TABLE OF CONTENTS

INTRODUCTION

Eating a decent diet and getting enough exercise are important to each individual's physical wellbeing and prosperity, yet they are especially important for individuals who must screen their kidneys' wellbeing.

When your kidneys are working ordinarily, they help you control the supplements and minerals moving through your body. If you have a kidney infection, your kidneys are normally not carrying out this activity correctly. To ensure that you get the correct proportion of protein, calories, nutrients, and minerals (and, as much as possible, the development of waste in your circulatory system), your doctor will, in all likelihood, suggest that carefully plan your diet.

How you deal with your diet will depend upon numerous variables. Patients who are on dialysis, for example, can have different needs from somebody who is in the beginning period of chronic kidney disease. Other ailments (diabetes, hypertension, excess weight, and so forth) can have further influences.

These and a few different features are examined in this book.

CHAPTER 1
THE RENAL DIET

WHAT IS A "RENAL DIET"?

A renal diet is essentially a diet that has been recommended for somebody with kidney disease. It depends on the phase of kidney disease, blood work results, drugs, and other dietary needs. However, because there is no standard renal diet, the diet can change from individual to individual and over time. The objectives of the diet are many in number and include the following:

- To prevent the development of poisons that kidneys typically get out of the blood
- To lessen the outstanding tasks that the kidneys must complete (before dialysis)
- To prevent complexities that can arise due to poisons
- To meet dietary needs

While the diet might be different for everybody, most followers are confined to sodium, potassium, phosphorus, and low or high protein needs. A few people may require a liquid diet. A registered dietitian will devise a care plan that is individualized to meet your particular needs.

At the point when you have chronic kidney disease, diet is a significant aspect of your treatment plan. Your prescribed diet may change after time if your kidney disease deteriorates. Not every person has similar restrictions and everybody's diet is individualized. Supplements influencing the kidneys are protein, sodium, potassium, and phosphorus.

Protein

- Eating the perfect amount of protein will help to construct muscles and fix tissues, battle contaminants, and maintain the structure of your blood.
- Large amounts of protein can burden the kidney – keep portions to 3 ounces for each serving.
- Protein is found in red meats, poultry (chicken, turkey, duck), fish and other seafood, eggs, milk, cheese, tofu, vegetables, and beans.

Tip: There are two types of protein. The best protein originates from animal-based items like meat, poultry, fish, eggs, and dairy. These are the most effortless proteins for your body to use.

Lower quality protein originates from vegetables and grains. A well-adjusted diet should include the two sorts of proteins consistently.

Sodium

- Limiting sodium (a mineral found in many foods) to 2000-3000 mg per day lessens the development of liquid in the body and controls circulatory strain.
- Sodium is found in many foods but is particularly high in:
- Table salt and ocean salt
- Salty seasonings (for example, soy sauce, teriyaki sauce, garlic salt, and flavoring salt)
- Most canned foods and some frozen foods – prepared meats (for example, ham, bacon, hotdogs, and cold cuts)
- Salted snack foods (for example, chips, saltines, and pickles)
- Most restaurant and take-out foods – canned or dried soups (for example, packaged noodle soup)

Tips:

- Eat foods nearest to their characteristic state (natural).
- Read food labels for sodium content.
- Try fresh or dried herbs and flavors rather than table salt.

- Provide flavor with hot pepper sauce. Vinegar, lemon juice, oils, and flavors can be used to marinate meat.
- Include salt mixes (Mrs. Dash®, McCormick's No Salt Added®)
- Keep away from salt substitutes (Half Salt® or No-Salt®)

Potassium

- Potassium is a significant mineral that helps your muscles and heart function well.
- A surplus or deficit of potassium in the blood can be dangerous.
- Not all people need the same amount of potassium.
- The amount you need will rely upon:
- How well your kidneys are functioning
- Whether you are taking certain kinds of drugs
- Potassium is found in all foods; large amounts are found in:
- Certain fruits and vegetables (bananas, melons, oranges, potatoes, tomatoes, dried fruits, dark green verdant vegetables, and some fruits and vegetable juices), milk and yogurt, dried beans and peas, salt substitutes, chocolate, nuts and seeds, lentils, and vegetables

Tip:

- Know your blood potassium level (typical 3.5-5.0).
- If it is too low, you may require a supplement to raise the level.
- If it is too high, you should avoid high-potassium foods.

Phosphorus

- Phosphorus is a mineral that works with calcium to form healthy bones and teeth.
- In kidney disease, phosphorus begins to develop in your blood. Calcium is pulled away from the bone and into the blood, causing significant issues like:
- Harm to the heart and different organs, poor blood flow, bone problems, skin ulcers
- Phosphorus is found in many foods. Large sums are found in:
- Dairy items (milk, cheddar cheese, pudding, yogurt, frozen yogurt)
- Dried beans and peas (kidney beans, split peas, lentils), nuts and seeds
- Different drinks (colas, brew, cocoa)
- Chocolate
- Whole grains, particularly wheat
- Prepared meats and fast foods
- Preparing powder

Tips:

- Use non-dairy flavors and suggested milk substitutes instead of milk to help bring down the amount of phosphorus in your diet.

EATING RIGHT FOR CHRONIC KIDNEY DISEASE

You must change what you eat to deal with your chronic kidney disease (CKD). Work with a registered dietitian to create a meal plan that includes foods that you like eating while at the same time maintaining your kidney's wellbeing.

The steps below will enable you to eat well as you deal with your kidney disease. The initial three stages (1-3) are significant for all individuals with kidney disease. The last two stages (4-5) may be significant as your kidney capacity decreases.

THE INITIAL STEPS TO EATING RIGHT

1. Choose and Prepare Foods With Less Salt and Sodium

Why? To help control your circulatory strain. Your diet should contain under 2,300 milligrams of sodium every day.

- Buy new food regularly. Sodium (a type of salt) is added to many packaged foods you purchase at the grocery or restaurant.
- Cook your own food instead of eating fast food or packaged foods that have lots of sodium.
- Use flavors, herbs, and no-sodium seasonings instead of salt.
- Check for sodium on the nutrition facts. A daily value of 20% or more means that the food is high in sodium.
- Try lower-sodium variants of pre-packaged or convenience foods.
- Wash canned vegetables, beans, meats, and fish with water before eating.

Search for food labels with words like sodium-free or salt-free; low, decreased, or no salt or sodium; or unsalted or lightly salted.

A food that has a daily value of 5% or less is low in sodium. Likewise, search for the amount of immersed and trans-fats on the label.

2. Eat the Perfect Amount and the Correct Kinds of Protein

Why? To help your kidneys. If you consume too much protein, it goes to waste that your kidneys evacuate. Consuming more protein than you need may make your kidneys work more than necessary.

- Consume small portions of protein-rich foods.
- High amounts of protein can be found in foods from animals and plants. A great many people eat the two kinds of protein. Talk with your dietitian about how to pick the correct mix of protein foods for you.

Animal-protein foods:

- Chicken
- Fish
- Meat
- Eggs
- Dairy

A cooked serving of chicken, fish, or meat is around 2 to 3 ounces, or about the size of a deck of cards. A serving of dairy foods is ½ cup of milk or yogurt, or one cut of cheddar.

Plant-protein foods:

- Beans
- Nuts
- Grains

A serving of cooked beans is about ½ cup, while a serving of nuts is ¼ cup. A serving of bread is a solitary cut, while a serving of cooked rice or cooked noodles is ½ cup.

3. Choose Foods That Are Sound for Your Heart

Why? To help prevent fat from building up in your veins, heart, and kidneys.

- Grill, sear, heat, dish, or pan-fry foods.
- Cook with nonstick cooking oil or a limited quantity of olive oil rather than margarine.
- Reduce fat from meat and peel skin from poultry before eating it.
- Try to avoid saturated and trans fats. Look at the food labels.

Heart-healthy foods:

- Lean cuts of meat, for example, midsection or round
- Poultry without the skin
- Fish
- Beans
- Vegetables
- Fruits
- Low-fat or no-fat milk, yogurt, and cheddar

Liquor

Drink liquor with restraint – one beverage per day if you are female, and two beverages per day if you are male. Drinking an excessive amount of liquor can harm the liver, heart, and mind and cause severe medical issues. Ask your doctor how much liquor you can drink safely.

The Subsequent Stages to Eating Right

As your kidney capacity decreases, you may need to eat foods with less phosphorus and potassium. Your doctor will use laboratory tests to check the potassium and phosphorus levels in your blood. Then you can work with your dietitian to change your meal plan.

4. Choose Foods and Beverages With Less Phosphorus

Why? To help protect your bones and veins. When you have CKD, phosphorus can develop in your blood. An excessive amount of phosphorus in your blood pulls calcium away from your bones, making them slim, frail, and bound to break. Significant levels of phosphorus in your blood can also cause irritated skin and bone and joint problems.

- Many packaged foods have included phosphorus. Search for phosphorus—or for words with "PHOS"— on fixing marks.

- Deli meats and some fresh meats and poultry can have phosphorus. Request that the butcher help you pick fresh meats without phosphorus.

Foods Lower in Phosphorus:

- Fresh vegetables
- Bread, pasta, rice
- Rice milk
- Corn and rice grains
- Light-colored soft drinks/pop, for example, lemon-lime

Foods Higher in Phosphorus:

- Meat, poultry, fish
- Bran grains and oats
- Dairy foods
- Beans, lentils, nuts
- Dark-colored soft drinks/pop, fruit juice, some packaged or canned sweet teas that have phosphorus

Your health-care provider may talk to you about taking a phosphate fastener with dinners to lower the amount of phosphorus in your blood. A phosphate folio is a medication that absorbs, or ties, phosphorus while it is in the stomach. Because it is bound, the phosphorus doesn't get into your blood. Rather, your body expels the phosphorus through your stool.

5.   *Choose Foods With the Perfect Amount of Potassium*

Why? To support your nerves and muscles. Issues can arise when your blood potassium levels are excessively high or excessively low. Unhealthy kidneys enable potassium to develop in your blood, which can cause heart issues. The foods you eat and the beverages you drink can help decrease your potassium level, if necessary.

- Salt substitutes can be high in potassium. Check with your supplier about using salt substitutes.
- Drain canned vegetables before consuming them.

Foods Lower in Potassium:

- Apples, peaches
- Carrots, green beans
- White bread, pasta
- White rice
- Rice milk
- Cooked rice and wheat oats, cornmeal
- Apple, grape, or cranberry juice

Foods Higher in Potassium:

- Oranges, bananas, and orange juice
- Potatoes, tomatoes
- Brown and wild rice
- Oat bran
- Dairy foods
- Whole-wheat bread and pasta
- Beans and nuts

A few medications can raise your potassium level. Your doctor may change the medications you take.

CHAPTER 2
7-DAY SAMPLE RENAL DIET MEAL PLAN

For individuals with diabetes and kidney disease, it is important to follow a diet that meets your individual needs.

Before following this plan, consult a registered dietitian.

MONDAY

Breakfast:

- 1 cup oatmeal
- ½ cup raspberries
- ½ cup milk or Rice Dream

Lunch:

- 1 pita pocket with
- 3 oz. chicken, salmon, leftover pork souvlaki
- ½ cup celery sticks and cut peppers
- 1 apple

Dinner:

- Onion-smothered steak
- 1 cup squashed potatoes

- ½ cup green beans
- 1 teaspoon margarine
- ½ cup mixed greens and 1 tablespoon dressing

Snack:

- 4 cups air-popped popcorn
- 3 teaspoons margarine

TUESDAY

Breakfast:

- 2 pieces toast
- 1 poached egg
- ½ cup blueberries
- 2 teaspoons margarine

Lunch:

- Turkey and pasta salad
- ½ cup pineapple
- ½ cup milk

Dinner:

- Flame-broiled fish in foil
- 1 cup rice
- 1 teaspoon margarine
- Flame-broiled corn on the cob or 1 cup popcorn

Snack:

- 1 renal-friendly whole-grain muffin
- 2 teaspoons margarine

WEDNESDAY

Breakfast:

- 3 low-phosphorus pancakes with syrup
- ½ cup strawberries
- 3 tablespoons whipping cream

Lunch:

- 1 burger bun
- 2 oz. leftover cut steak
- 1 teaspoon mustard
- 1 cup mixed greens/1 tablespoon dressing
- 1 cup vegetable stock
- ½ cup watermelon

Dinner:

- 1 serving cranberries
- Spare ribs
- 1 cup potato salad

Snack:

- 1 piece of toast/bread with margarine
- 1 ounce cheddar cheese

THURSDAY

Breakfast:

- ½ cup Special K
- 2 pieces of toast
- 1 tablespoon nutty spread
- ½ cup canned peaches
- ½ cup milk or Rice Dream

Lunch:

- 2 ounces leftover spareribs
- 1 dinner roll with 2 teaspoons margarine
- ½ cup coleslaw
- 1 mandarin orange

Dinner:

- 3 ounces herbed chicken
- 1 cup potatoes with 2 teaspoons margarine
- 1 cup green peas with 1 teaspoon margarine

Snack:

- 2 rice cakes with 2 teaspoons margarine and jam

FRIDAY

Breakfast:

- 1½ cups Cream of Wheat
- ½ cup blueberries
- ½ cup milk or Rice Dream

Lunch:

- Linguine with garlic and shrimp
- ½ cup fruit cocktail

Dinner:

- Meat and barley stew
- 1 piece of bread
- 1 cup mixed greens
- 2 tablespoons dressing

Snack:

- 2 cups air-popped popcorn
- 1½ teaspoon margarine

SATURDAY

Breakfast:

- Vegetable omelet
- 3 hash brown patties

Snack:

- Blueberry-lemon muffin
- 1 mandarin orange
- 1 teaspoon margarine

Dinner:

- Cooked red pepper pizza
- ½ cup salad
- 1 tablespoon dressing

Snack:

- 1 cup cornflakes
- 1 medium apple
- ½ cup milk

SUNDAY

Breakfast:

- 1 cup Cheerios
- 1 tangerine
- ½ cup milk or Rice Dream

Lunch:

- Leftover beef and barley stew
- 1 piece of bread
- 2 teaspoons margarine

Dinner:

- Pork souvlaki
- 1 cup rice
- 1 cup flame-broiled asparagus (12 lances)
- 2 teaspoons margarine
- ½ cup quick pear dessert

NOTES

Liquids:

- Limit coffee to 3 cups a day
- Limit tea to 5 cups a day
- Consume water throughout the day and during meals.

CHAPTER 3
FOODS TO DO AWAY WITH IF YOU HAVE BAD KIDNEYS

Your kidneys are bean-shaped organs that perform numerous important tasks.

The kidneys are responsible for separating blood, evacuating waste through urine, creating hormones, and adjusting minerals.

Many factors can cause kidney disease. Two of the most common are hypertension and uncontrolled diabetes.

Coronary illness, alcohol abuse, hepatitis C infection, and HIV contamination are additional causes.

When the kidneys are damaged and can't work properly, liquid can develop in the body and waste can collect in the blood.

Therefore, staying away from, or limiting your consumption, of certain foods may help reduce waste products in the blood, improve your kidney capacity, and avoid further harm.

THE CONNECTION BETWEEN RENAL DIET AND KIDNEY DISEASE

Dietary limitations change based on the phase of kidney disease.

For instance, individuals who in the beginning stages of chronic kidney disease will different dietary needs in comparison to those with end-stage renal disease.

Patient who have end-stage renal disease and who need dialysis will also have fluctuating dietary requirements. Dialysis is a treatment that removes excess liquid from the body.

Many of those in the late stages of kidney disease should follow a kidney-accommodating diet to avoid the development of substances in the blood.

For those with chronic kidney disease, the kidneys can't enough expel enough potassium, phosphorus, and sodium. Consequently, they're at a greater risk of increased amounts of those minerals in the blood.

A kidney-accommodating diet, or a "renal diet," as a rule limits sodium and potassium to 2,000 mg per day and restricts phosphorus to 1,000 mg daily.

Affected kidneys may also experience difficulty separating the waste resulting from protein digestion. Subsequently, people with chronic kidney disease in stages 1–4 may need to limit the amount of protein in their diets.

However, those with end-stage renal disease who are experiencing dialysis will need more protein.

Here are seventeen (17) foods that you should probably stay away from when on a renal diet.

1. Dark-Colored Colas

In addition to calories and sugar, colas contain added substances with phosphorus, particularly dark-colored colas.

Many food makers include phosphorus during the preparation of food and drinks to lengthen the product's lifespan.

This additional phosphorus is substantially more absorbable by the human body than regular, meat-based, or plant-based phosphorus.

In contrast to regular phosphorus, phosphorus as an added substance isn't bound to protein. Or it's found as a salt and can be easily absorbed by the intestinal tract.

Added phosphorus can ordinarily be found in an item's label. However, food makers are not required to list the precise amount of added phosphorus on the label.

Most dark-colored colas contain 50–100 mg of phosphorus in a 200-ml serving.

However, one should stay away from dark-colored colas when on a renal diet.

Synopsis: Dark-colored colas should be avoided on a renal diet because they contain added phosphorus, which is exceptionally permeable by the body's cells.

2. Avocados

These are frequently touted for their numerous nutritious characteristics, including their heart-sound fats, fiber, and cell reinforcements.

While avocados are normally a sound addition to a diet, people with kidney disease may have to avoid them.

This because avocados are rich in potassium. One cup (150 grams) of avocado contains an astounding 727 mg of potassium.

That is twice the amount of potassium in a medium banana.

Consequently, avocados, including guacamole, should be avoided on a renal diet, especially if you have been advised to watch your potassium consumption.

Avocados should be avoided on a renal diet because of their high potassium content. One cup of avocado contains about 37% of the 2,000 mg potassium limit.

3. Canned Foods

Canned foods like soups, vegetables, and beans are frequently consumed because they are easy to prepare.

However, most canned foods contain a lot of sodium, as salt is used as a preservative.

As a result, it's regularly advised that individuals with kidney disease should stay away from or limit their consumption of canned foods.

Picking lower-sodium options or those marked "no salt included" is normally best.

Moreover, rinsing canned foods, for example, canned beans and fish, can diminish the sodium content by 33–80%, based upon the item.

Synopsis

Canned foods are frequently high in sodium (Na). Avoiding low-sodium substances is a great step to decreasing your general sodium use.

4. Wheat Bread

Choosing the right bread can be difficult for people with kidney disease.

For healthy people, whole-wheat bread is typically preferred to over-refined, white flour bread.

Whole-wheat bread might be a nutritious decision because of its higher fiber content. However, white bread is normally preferred over whole-wheat options for people with kidney disease.

This is because of its potassium and phosphorus content. The more whole grains and wheat in the bread, the higher the potassium and phosphorus level.

Let's take, for example, a 30-gram serving of whole-wheat bread, which has about 69 mg of potassium and 57 mg of phosphorus. Meanwhile, white bread contains only 25 mg of both phosphorus and potassium.

Always keep in mind that most bread and bread items, regardless of whether they are white or whole-wheat, contain generally high amounts of sodium.

It's ideal to choose a lower-sodium alternative, if possible, and limit your portions.

Synopsis

White bread is normally preferred to wheat bread on a renal diet due to its lower potassium and phosphorus levels. As we all know, all bread contains sodium, so it's ideal to pick a lower-sodium choice.

5. Dark-Colored Rice

Like whole-wheat bread, dark-colored rice is a whole grain that has a higher phosphorus and potassium content than its white rice partner.

One cup of cooked dark rice contains 130 mg of phosphorus and 144 mg of potassium, while one cup of cooked white rice contains just 69 mg of phosphorus and 54 mg of potassium.

You might be able to fit dark rice into a renal diet if you limit the amount and offset it with different foods to limit your daily intake of phosphorus and potassium.

Buckwheat, bulgur, pearled grain, and couscous are nutritious, lower-phosphorus grains that can make a decent substitute for dark-colored rice.

Synopsis

Dark-colored rice is high in phosphorus and potassium and should be limited or avoided on a renal diet. White rice, bulgur, buckwheat, and couscous are great options.

6. Bananas

Bananas are known for their rich potassium (K) content.

Bananas are normally low in sodium; one medium banana contains 422 mg of potassium.

It can be hard to limit your everyday potassium intake to 1,500 mg.

Unfortunately, numerous other tropical fruits are high in potassium, too.

However, pineapples contain much less potassium than other tropical fruits, so they are a reasonable yet delicious choice.

Synopsis

Bananas are rich sources of potassium and should be restricted on a renal diet. As for pineapple, it is a kidney-accommodating fruit that contains significantly less potassium than other tropical fruits.

7. Dairy

Dairy items are plentiful in different nutrients and supplements.

In addition, dairy products are a good source of phosphorus and potassium as well as a good source of protein.

For instance, 1 cup (8 liquid ounces) of whole milk contains 222 mg of phosphorus and 349 mg of potassium.

However, consuming an excessive amount of dairy, related to different phosphorus-rich foods, can be damaging to the bone in those with kidney disease.

This may sound strange, as milk and dairy are frequently prescribed for healthy bones and muscle wellbeing.

However, when the kidneys are affected, lots of phosphorus can lead to an accumulation of phosphorus in the blood. This can make your bones thin and fragile after a while, leading to the risk of breakage or cracking.

Dairy items are also high in protein. One cup (8 liquid ounces) of whole milk contains around 8 grams of protein.

It might be necessary to restrict dairy consumption to avoid the accumulation of protein in the bloodstream.

Dairy products like almond milk and unenriched rice milk are a lot lower in phosphorus, potassium, and protein than cow's milk, making them a decent substitute for milk on a renal diet.

Synopsis

Dairy products contain high amounts of phosphorus, potassium, and protein and should be restricted on a renal diet. Regardless of milk's high calcium content, its phosphorus content may debilitate bones in those with kidney disease.

8. Orange Juice and Oranges

While orange juice and oranges are seemingly outstanding for their vitamin C content, they are also rich sources of potassium.

One large orange (184 grams) contains 333 mg of potassium. In addition, there is 473 mg of potassium in one cup (8 liquid ounces) of squeezed orange.

Due to their rich potassium content, orange juice and oranges should be avoided or restricted on a renal diet.

Apples, grapes, and cranberries, along with their individual juices, are, for the most part, great substitutes for oranges and orange juice, as they have lower potassium levels.

Synopsis

Oranges and orange juice are high in potassium and should be restricted on a renal diet. Instead, eat grapes, apples, cranberries, or their juices.

9. Prepared Meats

Prepared meats have for some time been related to chronic diseases and are commonly viewed as unhealthy because of their additives. Prepared meats are meats that have been salted, dried, preserved, or canned.

A few types include hot dogs, bacon, pepperoni, and jerky.

Prepared meats ordinarily contain a lot of salt, generally to improve taste and promote preservation.

Thus, it might be hard to keep your every-day sodium consumption to under 2,000 mg whenever prepared meats are included in your diet.

Also, prepared meats are high in protein.

If you have been advised to watch your protein consumption, it's imperative that you restrict your consumption of prepared meats.

Synopsis

Prepared meats are high in salt and protein and should be consumed with some restraint on a renal diet.

10. Pickles, Olives, and Relish

Pickles, prepared olives, and relish are, for the most part, examples of preserved or salted foods.

Generally, a lot of salt is added during the pickling process.

For instance, one pickle lance can contain in excess of 300 mg of sodium. Similarly, there is 244 mg of sodium in two tablespoons of sweet pickle relish.

Prepared olives will also, in general, be salty because they are preserved and aged. Five green salted olives contain around 195 mg of sodium, which is a significant amount of your daily serving.

Many stores stock low-sodium options for pickles, olives, and relish.

Synopsis

Pickles, prepared olives, and relish are high in sodium and should be restricted on a renal diet.

11. Apricots

Apricots are plentiful in vitamin C, nutrients, and fiber.

They are also high in potassium. One cup of new apricots contains 427 mg of potassium.

Moreover, dried apricots contain greater amounts of potassium.

One cup of dried apricots contains more than 1,500 mg of potassium.

This means that only one cup of dried apricots contains 75% of the 2,000 mg daily allotment.

It's ideal to stay away from apricots, and in particular dried apricots, on a renal diet.

Synopsis

Apricots are a high-potassium food that should be avoided on a renal diet. They contain over 400 mg for every 1 cup raw, and over 1,500 mg for every 1 cup dried.

12. Potatoes and Sweet Potatoes

Potatoes and sweet potatoes are potassium-rich vegetables.

Only one medium-sized prepared potato (156 g) contains 610 mg of potassium, while one normal sweet potato (114 g) contains 541 mg of potassium.

Luckily, some high-potassium foods, including potatoes and sweet potatoes, can be drenched or filtered to decrease their potassium content.

Cutting potatoes into small pieces and boiling them for 10 minutes can diminish the potassium content by about half.

Potatoes that are boiled in a large pot of water for four hours before cooking are known to have an even lower potassium content than those not boiled before cooking.

This strategy is known as "potassium filtering," or the "twofold cook technique."

While twofold cooking potatoes lowers the potassium content, it's critical to remember that this strategy doesn't completely eliminate the potassium.

Extensive amounts of potassium can be found in twofold cooked potatoes, so it's ideal to practice portion control to keep potassium levels within proper limits.

Synopsis

Potatoes and sweet potatoes are high-potassium vegetables. Boiling or twofold cooking potatoes can diminish potassium by about half.

13. Tomatoes

Tomatoes are another high-potassium natural product that may not fit the rules of a renal diet.

They can be served raw or stewed and are frequently used to make sauces.

Only one cup of tomato sauce can contain as much as 900 mg of potassium.

Unfortunately, for those on a renal diet, tomatoes are normally used in numerous dishes.

Picking an option with lower potassium content depends to a great extent on taste. However, swapping tomato sauce for a broiled red pepper sauce can be a good idea, all while providing less potassium per serving.

Synopsis

Tomatoes are another high-potassium organic product that should probably be restricted on a renal diet.

14. Packaged, Instant, and Pre-Made Meals

Prepared foods can account for a significant portion of sodium in a diet.

Among these foods, packaged, instant, and pre-made suppers are typically the most vigorously prepared and, thus, contain the most sodium.

Examples include frozen pizza, microwaveable suppers, and instant noodles.

Keeping sodium consumption to 2,000 mg per day might be difficult if you are eating processed foods all the time.

Not only do processed foods contain a lot of sodium, but they are generally low in supplements, too.

Synopsis

Packaged, instant, and pre-made suppers can contain a lot of sodium and supplements. It's ideal to restrict these foods on a renal diet.

15. Swiss Chard, Spinach, and Beet Greens

Swiss chard, spinach, and beet greens are verdant green vegetables that contain high amounts of supplements and minerals, including potassium.

When served raw, the amount of potassium shifts between 140–290 mg per cup.

While verdant vegetables shrink to a smaller serving size when cooked, the potassium content continues as before.

For instance, a half-cup of raw spinach will shrink to around one tablespoon when cooked. In this way, a half cup of cooked spinach will contain a lot more potassium than a half-cup of raw spinach.

To avoid a lot of potassium, consume a moderate amount of raw Swiss chard, spinach, and beet greens instead of consuming cooked greens.

Synopsis

Verdant green vegetables like Swiss chard, spinach, and beet greens are brimming with potassium, particularly when served cooked. In spite of the fact that serving size decreases when cooked, potassium content remains as before.

16. Dates, Raisins, and Prunes

Dates, raisins, and prunes are regular dried fruits.

When fruits are dried, the majority of their supplements are concentrated, including potassium.

For instance, one cup of prunes contains 1,274 mg of potassium, which is many times greater than the amount of potassium found in one cup of its raw partner, plums.

Additionally, only four dates contain 668 mg of potassium.

Given the amazing amount of potassium in these basic dried fruits, it's ideal to avoid them while on a renal diet to guarantee that your potassium levels remain ideal.

Synopsis

Supplements are concentrated when fruits are dried. Along these lines, the potassium content of dried organic fruit, including dates, prunes, and raisins, is incredibly high and should be avoided on a renal diet.

17. Pretzels, Chips, and Crackers

Prepared nibble foods like pretzels, chips, and saltines will, in general, be deficient in supplements and moderately high in salt.

Additionally, it's easy to eat more than the prescribed serving size of these foods, frequently leading to more salt consumption than planned.

In addition, if chips are made from potatoes, they will contain a lot of potassium.

Synopsis

Pretzels, chips, and wafers are often consumed in large portions and will, in general, contain high amounts of salt. Also, chips produced using potatoes contain a lot of potassium.

CHAPTER 4
GETTING MORE ENERGY FROM KIDNEY-FRIENDLY FOODS

Your energy level doesn't need to go down just because the sun does. You can have energy for the duration of the day, even after work or a dialysis treatment. It might be simpler than you suspect.

To Getting Healthy, Eat Foods on the Kidney Diet

What you eat extraordinarily influences your energy level. Suppers that are excessively high in refined starches and low in protein may cause a brisk increase in glucose, trailed by a similarly fast drop, which makes you feel less energetic only an hour or two later. However, a well-adjusted and kidney-accommodating supper with sound starches (fruits, vegetables, and healthy grains) combined with a decent source of protein (fish, poultry, egg whites, lean meat, protein powder, or a supplement) can help keep maintain glucose levels and keep you alert.

Timing Is Everything When You Need Energy

The time when you eat is a factor in how your energy level is managed. Skipping dinners will decrease your energy level. Because food fuels all movement—both physical and mental—you'll experience considerable difficulties working if your tank is vacant. If you avoid dinner, you'll likely be enticed to get the fastest food possible. If you stop at a drive-through, the food will be less nutritious. If you are in a hurry when you have to eat, try to stay away from overly prepared foods stacked with sodium and phosphorus – for example, packaged foods.

Plan to keep sound snacks around – for example, low-potassium leafy foods, grains and easy-to-get sources of protein. If you need a hearty dinner, a protein bar can be used as a substitute. Talk to your dietitian about which protein bars are suitable for your kidney diet.

Exercise, the Kidney Diet, and Energy

Wellness is another factor that determines how much energy you have for the duration of the day. Individuals who are fit will use energy all the more productively; accordingly, they have more energy to get them through the day.

Some individuals with chronic kidney disease (CKD) may state that they feel too worn out to even think about exercising. However, to avoid fatigue, you'll want to keep moving. At the point when your energy is slacking, ordinary exercise can prompt better and more tranquil rest, which means you will store up more energy to use the following day. It might sound odd, but the more you work out, the more energy you'll have.

Eat, Practice, and Invigorate

Realizing what to eat and when to eat it alongside better wellness can be the formula for having more energy. You'll achieve your objectives all the more successfully, which leaves you time for other things.

For some individuals on dialysis, exhaustion and low energy are typical side effects. This drowsiness might be the result of numerous factors, including the foods in an individual's diet. What and when we eat can affect energy levels and execution for the duration of the day. Other dietary causes of weakness can include an excessive amount of liquor, an absence of specific nutrients, iron insufficiency, frailty, or a lack of food. Certain diseases, drugs, stress, or inadequate rest can add to fatigue, also. Fortunately, individuals can streamline their body's potential by consuming a well-adjusted kidney diet that lifts energy from sun up to sun down and improves personal satisfaction.

Our bodies get energy from the foods we eat and drink. Foods containing sugars, proteins, and fats provide calories that are used by our bodies to deliver energy. The amount of calories we need relies upon our age, size, sexual orientation, physical activity level, and health status. In this manner, eating the perfect amount of calories throughout the day can help individuals have energy exactly when they need it. Renal dietitians help dialysis patients decide on the number of calories and protein they need every day to upgrade their energy levels.

To get enough energy from kidney-accommodating foods, dialysis patients must include foods rich in starches, proteins, and fat.

Kidney-Accommodating Starches and Energy

Starches are the body's favored energy source. In line with this, the most ideal approach to boost the body's potential is to eat sugar-rich foods. Complex carbs – for example, rice, pasta, and dark vegetables – are high in sugars, a portion of which contain fiber. They also provide a consistent source of glucose for energy and blood glucose. If an individual on dialysis has diabetes, spreading out starches for the duration of the day will help control glucose and boost energy. The key is to have the same amount of starches at every meal. The planning of suppers is profoundly linked to an individual's energy levels. Skipping suppers or eating dinners too far apart may negatively affect energy balance.

However, some starch-rich foods, for example, vegetables and milk, are high in phosphorus and potassium. Individuals with kidney disease who need to control those supplements may need to restrict certain foods. Taking phosphate fasteners with every supper, in addition to working with a dietitian to help make good food decisions, can help balance phosphorus and potassium in an individual's dialysis diet.

Kidney-Accommodating Proteins and Energy

Foods rich in protein also help streamline the utilization of energy in our bodies. Eating the perfect amount of protein is particularly significant for patients on dialysis. During the dialysis treatment, some protein is lost; a lack of protein can affect the immune system, impede healing, and result in unbalanced hormones. Maintaining your protein stores by consuming the perfect amount of protein and calories will enable you to feel your best. The amount of protein an individual needs relies upon numerous variables, for example, body size, activity level, and dialysis medicines. Renal dietitians counsel patients on how much protein they need. Great sources of protein are lean meats, including eye of round hamburger, lean ground meat, pork tenderloin, poultry, fish, eggs, and egg substitutes. Because numerous protein-rich foods are also high in phosphorus, taking phosphate covers before or with your suppers will help keep phosphorus in check. Consider consuming two ounces of high-protein food or taking a protein supplement that contains roughly 14 grams of protein during every dialysis treatment. This will help replace protein lost during treatment.

Kidney-Accommodating Fats and Energy

Fats are a concentrated source of energy, and while they have an awful reputation, individuals need fat in their diet to perform at an optimal level. In addition to giving us energy, fats keep us warm and help us use certain nutrients. Consuming too much fat can prompt weight increase and coronary illness. There are two sorts of fats: saturated and unsaturated. Saturated fats, otherwise called bad fats, originate from animal-based foods, can raise cholesterol levels, and boost the threat of coronary illness. A few examples include hydrogenated cooking oils and prepared meats like bacon, hot dogs, and pepperoni. Restricting these high-fat foods on a kidney diet and choosing more unsaturated fats, otherwise called good fats, is a healthy method. Unsaturated fats include non-hydrogenated vegetable oils like canola, olive, or corn oil, and trans-fat-free margarine. Unsaturated fats help decrease cholesterol and provide additional energy. However, control is the key because too much of the good stuff can prompt undesirable weight gain and other medical issues.

Energy-Boosting Plans for the Kidney Diet

These dietitian-chosen plans will help kick off your day and maintain your energy.

Breakfast:

- Egg and Sausage Breakfast Sandwich
- Great Way to Start Your Day Bagel
- Raised Waffles

Lunch:

- Chicken Teriyaki Pita Sandwich
- Super Burgers
- Tuna Salad Bagel

Snacks:

- Easy Summer Fruit Dip
- Shrimp Spread with Crackers
- Spicy Crunch and Munch Snack Mix

Dinner:

- Baked Pork Chops
- Braised Short Ribs of Beef
- Cilantro Lime Cod

Energy from Your Kidney Diet

If an individual with kidney disease feels drowsy in spite of eating a decent amount of calories, starches, proteins, and fat, they should visit their primary care physician. Dialysis patients who want to eat the best assortment of foods will feel increasingly powerful if they make healthy kidney-accommodating food decisions for the duration of the day.

WEIGHT-LOSS DIETING WHEN YOU'RE ON DIALYSIS

If you are thinking about starting to eat better to get in shape, you may consider how to do so while following your dialysis diet. As with most diets, getting in shape on a dialysis diet can be difficult. If you diet correctly by eating right, working with your renal dietitian, and incorporating physical activity into your daily schedule, you can lose the undesirable pounds and feel more energetic.

Why a Few People on Dialysis Need to Get in Shape

If you are overweight and on dialysis, you may profit from weight reduction for the following reasons:

- Better glucose control if you have diabetes
- Better circulatory control
- Decreased cholesterol and triglyceride levels
- Increased energy
- Qualification for a kidney transplant

Step-by-Step Guide on How to Begin a Weight Reduction Diet When You're on Dialysis

There are a few things to know before you start any weight-reduction plan. At the point when you're on dialysis, talking with your dietitian and specialist about changes in your standard diet is important. Your dietitian can help you to create a meal plan that considers both your dialysis diet and your desire to get more fit, while your primary care physician may recommend which exercises are best for you. Tell them your objectives so you get the right advice for your weight reduction diet.

Following are weight reduction diet tips for individuals on dialysis:

- **Know about your shopping and dietary patterns**

- Keep a diary of the food you eat, your feelings, and your cravings.
- Don't skip suppers; this regularly results in gorging later on.
- Avoid interruptions while you eat – for example, watching TV during supper.
- Avoid snacking while planning suppers.
- Eat gradually.
- Don't shop for food when you're hungry.
- Before shopping for food, make a list and stick to it.

- **Exercise with your primary care physician's approval**

- Start gradually and limit your efforts to 30 minutes per day.
- Choose an action you like, for example, bicycling, swimming, or walking.
- Buy a pedometer to follow your steps; try to get in 10,000 steps per day.
- Take the stairs rather than the elevator.
- Park farther away from stores so you get in additional exercise while running errands.
- Ask about activities you can do in your seat if you can't get up.
- Monitor the calories you consume. Try using the Calorie Burn Tools to determine how many calories you consume.

- **Minimize calorie and fat consumption**

- Try diverse cooking strategies. Utilize a nonstick cooking dish. Additionally, cook in a way that won't add more fat to a meal, for example, by flame broiling.
- Choose lean cuts of hamburger, pork, sheep, and veal. Cut back the excess before cooking.
- Take the skin off poultry before cooking.

- Buy water-pressed canned fish, chicken, or different meats. Purchase low-sodium foods when available or wash them under cool water to eliminate excess sodium.
- Substitute low-fat mayonnaise for salad dressing.
- If you use nondairy creamers, search for the one with the least calories.
- Select graham crackers, low-fat treats, and vanilla wafers, rather than cakes, pies, doughnuts, or high-fat treats.
- Use sugar substitutes rather than normal sugar.
- Avoid iced oats or those with nuts. Try Corn Flakes, Rice Krispies, puffed rice, and other lower-calorie cereals.
- Substitute fresh foods for high-fat foods. Make sure to keep inside your potassium limit.
- Increase your fiber consumption to 25 grams per day. Approach your dietitian for tips on the best high-fiber foods to eat.

- **Be mindful of your portion sizes**

- Weigh or measure foods until you get a precise feeling for serving sizes.
- Portions should be the correct size.

Find the guidelines below:

- Carbs (grains, starches) = 1 cup (size of an adult fist)
- Protein (meat, fish, poultry) = 3 ounces (size of the palm of your hand)
- Fats (salad dressing, butter, etc.) = 1 teaspoon (size of a thumb tip)
- Vegetables and fruits = 1/2 cup (size of a little fist)
- Buy single-serve or smaller packages if you are enticed to eat more than one serving.
- When eating out, share a dinner or take half home.
- Use a dinner plan to decide what number of servings from every food group to incorporate every day.

- **Reward yourself**

At the point when you set sensible objectives and accomplish them, reward yourself. Here are a few recommendations:

- Go to the cinema.
- Buy an outfit, book, or CD.
- Have a bowling night with friends.

- *Troubles when attempting to shed weight on dialysis*

Weight loss can be difficult. It requires some investment and devotion to accomplish your weight-loss objectives. The challenges you may face are both physical and mental. Here are a few reasons why dialysis patients might be dissuaded from eating right and working out.

- *Physical*

Iron deficiency

A few people with chronic kidney disease (CKD) who are on dialysis have an iron deficiency because of a low red platelet count, which causes exhaustion, shortness of breath, and lightheadedness. Your primary care physician will create a treatment plan that will help treat iron deficiency. If you are sick, request that your primary care physician tell you when your blood count is sufficiently high.

After-treatment influences

Some dialysis patients who do in-focus hemodialysis can feel frail after treatment and therefore not be inspired to work out. This might last for only a few hours, or you may require a decent night's rest. Plan to exercise a few hours after treatment or on non-dialysis days.

Peritoneal dialysis (PD)

Individuals on peritoneal dialysis (PD) may experience difficulty shedding pounds because they retain glucose (sugar) from the dialysis. The glucose taken in during dialysis can, in some cases, equal as much as 500 calories per day. The best approach to avoiding weight gain while on peritoneal dialysis is to use dialysis arrangements with a minimal amount of glucose. That means using more 1.5% and 2.5% (yellow) packs and fewer 4.25% (red) packs. If this results in the retention of liquid, work with your dietitian and PD medical caretaker to determine the amount of salt and fluids you should consume every day.

Individuals on PD ordinarily have the opportunity and capacity to exercise, and this should be a part of your everyday schedule or program. A few people think that it is easier to exercise on an empty stomach as opposed to a full. This should be discussed with your doctor.

Sufficient protein

Decreasing food consumption, as a rule, cuts into the amount of protein eaten. If quality protein consumption is lacking when you are dieting, you may lose bulk and your albumin level may drop. Your dietitian can help ensure that you eat enough low-fat, quality protein. Dietitians can also screen your month-to-month labs to ensure your albumin isn't dropping.

- *Emotional*

Food decisions

In some cases, individuals make poor food decisions because of their emotions and indulge when they feel down, or even when they're upbeat and need to celebrate.

- *Staying on track*

Keep in mind that getting in shape won't happen without any forethought. Attempting to roll out gigantic improvements all at once can be debilitating. Set small objectives that can add up to a large achievement.

Talk to your dietitian about various meal plans that fit your objectives and way of life. Your dietitian may also acquaint you with frozen dinner that cut cooking time yet are low in phosphorus and potassium. Be sure to remove unnecessary calories – for example, high-fat and high-sugar foods. If you end up getting thinner so that you can join the transplant list, this demonstrates that you are so dedicated to your wellbeing.

Individuals who are effective at getting fit typically embrace the following habits:

- Keep a food journal.
- Eat balanced meals.

- Set realistic objectives.
- Include daily exercise.

Synopsis

Weight loss dieting when you're on dialysis can be an additional test. Getting fit doesn't happen without any forethought and it requires a great deal of devotion. Progressive changes may enable you to accomplish better outcomes. The methodology isn't only an adjustment in your diet; it also an adjustment in your way of life. You may end up being an example of overcoming adversity.

WEIGHT LOSS TIPS FOR THOSE WITH KIDNEY DISEASE

As explained in the previous chapter, shedding pounds might be hard work, yet it shouldn't be confusing. Individuals will, in general, underestimate the amount they really eat, which can add to weight gain. For those with kidney disease, certain dietary limitations add another component to the battle. It's not all bad news, however. This book is here to enable you to win your fight with extra weight. Get yourself in tune with the best way to kick off your New Year's goals with these five straightforward weight loss tips.

Before beginning another diet or exercise program, check with your physician or health care provider.

- *Log it:* Try keeping a diary or food log of everything you eat and drink every day. Incorporate serving estimates so you can determine where and when you're indulging. Try using apps to figure out how many calories you're really taking in every day. If you are following a diet for kidney disease, make it a point to monitor potassium, phosphorus and sodium, as well as calories, sugars, protein, and fat. You can also look into food values online by visiting the USDA food tables.

- *Create an activity plan:* It's possible to remain energetic no matter what's going on with your schedule. Schedule your physical movement and it will be easier to stay with it. Expect to get 30 minutes of activity, five times a week. To determine how many calories you've consumed, use portable apps, websites, and graphs.

- *Make basic swaps:* Look at the fatty foods you like and try to bring down the calorie count. For instance, rather than frying, try cooking or flame broiling. Watch out for meals at parties – limit yourself to smaller portions and consume them less frequently, as they can be high in calories, sodium, and phosphorus.

- *Still hungry?* When dieting, if your stomach rumbles, you aren't full. Try eating foods that will fill you up without destroying your diet. Concentrate on foods that are low in calories and high in fulfillment. These will fill your stomach, which will prevent you from quickly getting hungry again. Low-salt saltines can give you the crunch you pine for without the higher-salt, higher-fat content of chips. High-fiber foods, for example, fresh fruits* and vegetables* (particularly those with seeds and skins) and low-salt/low-fat popcorn are a few examples. Four cups of popped popcorn (air-popped or micro-waved, without salt and fat) contain around 100 calories and can truly be filling. If you are on a restricted liquid diet, try saving a portion of your liquids to have with your treats. This can also help you feel satiated.

- **Slow down:** If you eat rapidly, odds are that the food isn't particularly fulfilling. Rather, search for alternatives, like leafy greens that require a lot of chewing. This can slow your pace of eating, thereby helping you eat less. Additionally, try to enjoy each bit.

- If you are following a low-potassium as well as low-phosphorus diet, try the following:

Low-potassium vegetables (1 cup serving size): chunk of iceberg lettuce, raw cabbage, cucumbers, cauliflower, onions, ringer peppers, radishes, celery, carrots, and Chinese pea pods.

Low-potassium fruits: grapes, apples, mandarin oranges, pineapple, pears, blueberries, strawberries (limit one cup a day), blackberries, raspberries, and new plums (limit two plums a day).

CALORIES: A GUIDE TO ADDING OR LIMITING THEM ON THE KIDNEY DIET

If you have Stage 3 or 4 chronic kidney disease (CKD), your nephrologist (kidney specialist) may encourage you to incorporate certain improvements into your diet. If you are not at a sound weight, the specialist may propose that you either gain or shed a couple of pounds, based upon your condition. Keeping up a healthy weight can help individuals with kidney disease control and prevent more medical issues. If you lose excess weight, circulatory strain and glucose levels generally improve. This may delay or reduce additional kidney disease. If individuals need to add calories to their diet, they can halt the process of muscle loss and acquire energy for regular exercises.

When making changes in a diet or way of life, studies have demonstrated that changing just one or two things at a time works best. Once they become habits, you can make more changes.

The foods we eat contain calories, which give us energy. There are calories in many foods; however, there are higher amounts in quick foods, sweets, and things like doughnuts, chips, and soft drinks.

Minimizing Calories on the Kidney Diet

Here are a few guidelines to help in minimizing calories:

- "Eat like a lord at breakfast, a sovereign at lunch, and a homeless person at dinner."
- Eat all more fresh fruits and vegetables.
- Eat a serving of mixed greens every day.
- Use low-fat or fat-free dressings.
- Have unbuttered popcorn.
- Eat standard suppers and snacks if you need them to control desires.
- Omit juices and soft drinks.
- Don't eat after 8:00 p.m.
- Use a smaller plate for your dinners.
- Share a dinner when eating in a restaurant.
- Eat only when you are hungry, not out of boredom.
- Increase your movement level to help burn calories.

Perusing names makes a difference. Search for these keywords for foods that are lower in calories:

- Baked
- Broiled
- Grilled
- In its own juice
- Non-fat or low-fat
- Lean
- Marinara
- Poached
- Roasted
- Stir-fried
- Steamed

Including Calories in the Kidney Diet

If you have to put on weight, your primary care physician and dietitian may suggest that you:

- Use "good" fats generously.
- Sauté foods in canola or olive oil.
- Add low-salt dressings to servings of mixed greens and vegetables.
- Add low-salt flavors to meats.
- Include a few snacks in addition to suppers.
- Consume drinks that contain calories.
- Combine cream cheese with mayonnaise and herbs and use as a vegetable dip.

- Spread cream cheese on wafers and top with jam.
- Treat yourself to a fatty treat every day if you don't have diabetes.

Following are foods that are generally higher in calories:

- Basted
- Buttered
- Crispy
- Fried
- In sauce
- Pan-fried
- Sautéed
- Smothered

Get some information about the kidney-accommodating ways you can add calories to your diet. For example, homemade sauce might be high in calories, but the packaged kind is high in sodium. Your dietitian may prescribe a kidney-accommodating nutrition drink or bar to give you additional calories.

Kidney Diet Recipes/Regimens

There are numerous plans that you can try. These plans are largely useful for kidney diets, and they are good for starch control, as well as renal and renal diabetic food plans.

LOWER CALORIE KIDNEY DIET RECIPES

- Ambrosia
- Carrot Casserole
- Cranberry-Apple Salad
- Egg in a Hole
- German Pancakes
- Ratatouille
- Low-Fat Heavenly Fruit Hash
- Vegetable Paella

HIGHER CALORIE KIDNEY DIET RECIPES

- Banana Pudding Dessert
- Breakfast Burrito
- Citrus Salmon
- Slow Cooker BBQ Beef
- Solidified Sugar Cookie Sandwiches
- Farm Chicken Pasta
- Stuffed French Toast
- Turkey Waldorf Salad

Avoiding or adding calories when you're on the kidney diet can be difficult. However, by using this book, you can settle on the best possible choices for your kidney diet. Your dietitian can also guide you in determining the number of calories you need every day so you can follow a healthy diet while living with kidney disease.

CHAPTER 5
DIET FOR ADVANCED CHRONIC KIDNEY DISEASE IN ADULTS

Why is Nutrition Important for Advanced Chronic Kidney Disease?

An individual may avoid or postpone some medical issues resulting from chronic kidney disease (CKD) by eating the correct foods and staying away from foods high in sodium, potassium, and phosphorus. Learning about calories, fats, proteins, and liquids is important for an individual with chronic kidney disease. Protein-rich foods, for example, meat and dairy items, separate into waste items that healthy kidneys expel from the blood.

As chronic kidney disease advances, your needs will change. A doctor may suggest that a patient with diminished kidney capacity choose foods cautiously.

What Do the Kidneys Do?

The kidneys expel extra water and wastes from the blood and make urine. They also balance the salts and minerals – for example, calcium, phosphorus, sodium, and potassium – that are in the blood. The kidneys also discharge hormones that help red platelets, control the pulse, and keep bones healthy.

What Are the Impacts Of CKD?

In CKD, the kidneys keep working, though not as they should. Wastes may develop so continuously that the body ends up used to having them in the blood. Salts containing phosphorus and potassium may rise to dangerous levels, causing heart and bone issues. Iron deficiency – i.e., a low amount of platelets – can result from CKD because the kidneys quit making enough erythropoietin, a hormone that causes bone marrow to make platelets. After months or years, CKD may advance to the point at which the individual needs a kidney transplant or standard blood separating medications called dialysis.

What Is Medicinal Nourishment Therapy (MNT)?

MNT is the use of nourishment, directed by a registered dietitian, to help advance a medicinal or wellbeing objective. A medicinal services supplier may refer a patient to a registered dietitian to help with the patient's food plan. Many protection arrangements spread MNT when prescribed by a doctor. Anyone who meets all the requirements for Medicare can take advantage of MNT from a registered dietitian if a doctor provides a referral demonstrating that the individual has diabetes or kidney disease.

One approach toward finding a certified dietitian is to contact the Academy of Nutrition and Dietetics at www.eatright.org and click on "Locate a Registered Dietitian." Users can enter their location or ZIP code for a rundown of dietitians in their area. An individual searching for dietary guidance to avoid kidney disease should click on "Renal (Kidney) Nutrition" in the "claim to fame" field. Dietitians who spend a significant amount of time assisting individuals with CKD are called renal dietitians.

Importance of Knowing About Calories for Somebody With Advanced CKD

As CKD advances, individuals frequently lose their appetite because they find that foods don't taste as good. Thus, they expend less calories – significant units of energy in food – and may lose an excessive amount of weight. Renal dietitians can help individuals with CKD find healthy approaches to adding calories to their diet if they are losing a lot of weight.

Importance of Knowing About Protein for Somebody with Advanced CKD

Protein is a basic component of any diet. Proteins help assemble and look after muscle, bone, skin, connective tissue, interior organs, and blood. They help battle disease and mend wounds. However, proteins also separate into waste items that must be expelled from the blood via the kidneys. Consuming more protein than the body needs may put additional weight on the kidneys and cause kidney capacity to decrease quicker.

Doctors indicate that individuals with CKD should eat moderate or decreased amounts of protein. However, limiting protein could prompt a lack of sustenance, so individuals with CKD should be cautious. The average American diet contains adequate protein. Learning about portion sizes can help individuals limit their protein consumption without jeopardizing their wellbeing.

What Is the Correct Meat Portion?

The vast majority of people with or without CKD can get the daily protein they require by consuming a two- to three-ounce serving of meat or a meat supplement. A two-ounce serving of meat is about the size of a deck of cards or the palm of an individual's hand.

A renal dietitian can help individuals find out about the amount and sources of protein in their diets. Animal-based protein in egg whites, cheese, chicken, fish, and red meat contains a greater amount of the basic supplements a body needs. With careful dinner planning, a well-adjusted vegetarian diet can also provide these supplements. A renal dietitian can help individuals with CKD make small modifications to their dietary patterns that can bring about critical protein decreases. For instance, individuals can decrease their protein consumption by making sandwiches using slender cuts of meat and by including lettuce, cucumber, apple, and different trimmings. The following table contains some higher-protein foods and recommendations for lower-protein choices that are better decisions for individuals with CKD who are attempting to limit their protein consumption.

Higher- and Lower-Protein Foods

Higher-Protein Foods:

- Halibut
- Ground beef
- Shrimp
- Salmon
- Tuna
- Chicken bosom
- Roasted chicken

Lower-Protein Foods:

- Chili con carne
- Beef stew
- Egg substitutes
- Tofu
- Imitation crab meat

When kidney capacity decays to the point where dialysis is necessary, patients should include more protein in their diets, as dialysis expels a lot of protein from the blood.

Importance of Knowing About Fat for Somebody with Advanced CKD

Everybody should think about fat sources because eating an inappropriate type of fat, and a lot of fat, can result in blocked veins and heart issues. Fat provides energy, helps produce hormone-like substances that direct the pulse and other cardiac capacities, and conveys fat-solvent nutrients. Everybody needs dietary fat; however, a few fats are more advantageous than others. Individuals with CKD are at a higher risk of heart failure or stroke. Thus, individuals with CKD should be particularly cautious about how dietary fat influences their heart wellbeing.

Individuals with CKD should talk with a dietitian about healthy and undesirable sources of fat. Saturated fats and trans-unsaturated fats can raise blood cholesterol levels and stop up veins. Saturated fats are found in animal products, for example, red meat, poultry, and whole milk. Trans-unsaturated fats are frequently found in packaged products like treats and cakes and in fried foods like doughnuts and French fries.

A dietitian can recommend sound approaches to including fat in one's diet, particularly if more calories are required. Vegetable oils – for example, corn or safflower oil, are more beneficial than animal-based fats. Hydrogenated vegetable oils should be avoided because they are high in trans-unsaturated fats. Monounsaturated fats like olives, nuts, and canola oils are sound options in contrast to animal-based fats. The table below demonstrates the sources of fats, separated into three types of fats that should be eaten less frequently and good fats that can be eaten more regularly.

Sources of Fats

Eat Less Often	Eat More Often

Saturated fats

- Red meat
- Poultry
- Whole milk
- Butter
- Lard

Trans-unsaturated fats

- Commercially prepared products
- French fries
- Doughnuts

Hydrogenated vegetable oils

- Margarine
- Shortening

Monounsaturated fats

- Corn oil
- Safflower oil
- Olive oil
- Peanut oil
- Canola oil

Importance of Knowing About Sodium for Somebody with Advanced CKD

A lot of sodium in an individual's diet can be destructive because it causes blood to retain liquid. Individuals with CKD should be mindful so as not to allow an excessive amount of liquid to develop in their bodies. This additional liquid increases circulatory strain as well as puts a strain on the heart and kidneys. A dietitian can help individuals discover approaches to lessen the amount of sodium in their diet. Food labels give data about the sodium content in food. The U.S. Food and Drug Administration says that healthy individuals should limit their daily sodium consumption to close to 2,300 mg, the amount found in one teaspoon of table salt. Individuals who are in danger of a coronary episode or stroke due to a condition like hypertension or kidney disease should limit their every-day sodium consumption to close to 1,500 mg. Choosing no-sodium or low-sodium food items will enable them to reach that goal.

Sodium is found in common table salt and numerous salty seasonings, like soy sauce and teriyaki sauce. Canned foods, some frozen foods, and most prepared meats have a lot of salt. Nibble foods, for example, chips and wafers, are also high in salt.

Seasonings, for example, lemon juice, without salt flavoring, as well as hot pepper sauce can help individuals lessen their salt consumption. Individuals with CKD should avoid salt substitutes that contain potassium – for example, Also Salt or Nu-Salt – because CKD limits the body's capacity to dispose of potassium from the blood. The table below gives some high-sodium foods and recommendations for low-sodium options that are more beneficial for individuals with any degree of CKD who have hypertension.

High- and Low-Sodium Foods

High-Sodium Foods:

- Salt
- Regular canned vegetables
- Hot dogs and canned meat
- Packaged rice with sauce
- Packaged noodles with sauce
- Frozen vegetables with sauce
- Frozen prepared suppers
- Canned soup
- Regular tomato sauce

Low-Sodium Foods:

- Salt herb seasonings
- Low-sodium canned foods
- Fresh, cooked meat
- Plain rice without sauce
- Plain noodles without sauce
- Fresh vegetables without sauce
- Frozen vegetables without sauce
- Homemade soup with fresh fixings
- Reduced-sodium tomato sauce
- Unsalted pretzels
- Unsalted popcorn

Importance of Knowing About Potassium for Somebody with Advanced CKD

Keeping the correct amount of potassium in the blood is fundamental. Potassium keeps the heart beating regularly and the muscles working correctly. Issues can arise when blood potassium levels are either excessively low or excessively high. Damaged kidneys enable potassium to develop in the blood, causing heart issues. Potassium is found in numerous leafy foods, for example, bananas, potatoes, avocados, and melons. Individuals with CKD may need to stay away from certain vegetables. Blood tests can show when potassium levels are in a better-than-average range. A renal dietitian can help individuals with CKD discover approaches to restricting the amount of potassium they eat. The potassium content of potatoes and different vegetables can be decreased by boiling them in water. The following table provides examples of some high-potassium foods and low-potassium choices for individuals with CKD.

High- and Low-Potassium Foods

High-Potassium Foods:

- Oranges and orange juice
- Melons
- Apricots
- Bananas
- Potatoes
- Tomatoes
- Sweet potatoes

Low-Potassium Alternatives:

- Plums
- Canned pears
- Cabbage
- Pineapple
- Apples and apple juice
- Cranberries and cranberry juice
- Blueberries, raspberries, strawberries

High-Potassium Foods:

- Cooked broccoli
- Cooked spinach
- Beans

Low-Potassium Alternatives:

- Boiled cauliflower

Importance of Knowing About Potassium for Somebody with Advanced CKD

Damaged kidneys permit phosphorus, a mineral found in numerous foods, to develop in the blood. Excessive phosphorus in the blood pulls calcium from the bones, making the bones weak and prone to breaking. A lot of phosphorus can also make the skin tingle. Some foods, for example, milk and cheese, dried beans, colas, canned sweet teas and lemonade, nuts, and nutty spreads are high in phosphorus. A renal dietitian can help individuals with CKD figure out how to restrict phosphorus in their diet.

As CKD advances, an individual may need to take a phosphate folio, for example, sevelamer hydrochloride (Renagel), lanthanum carbonate (Fosrenol), calcium acetic acid derivation (PhosLo), or calcium carbonate (Tums) to control the phosphorus in the blood. These medications help absorb, or tie, phosphorus while it is in the stomach. Because it is bound, the phosphorus doesn't get into the blood. Rather, it is expelled from the body in the stool.

The table below contains some high-phosphorus foods and recommendations for low-phosphorus choices that are more advantageous for individuals with CKD.

High- and Low-Phosphorus Foods

High-Phosphorus Foods:

- Dairy foods (milk, cheese, yogurt)
- Beans (heated, kidney, lima, pinto)
- Nuts and nutty spreads
- Processed meats (franks, canned meat)
- Cola
- Canned sweet teas and lemonade
- Oat bran
- Egg yolks

Low-Phosphorus Alternatives:

- Liquid non-dairy flavor
- Sherbet
- Cooked rice
- Rice, wheat, and corn oats
- Popcorn
- Lemon-lime pop
- Root beer
- Powdered sweet tea and lemonade blends

Importance of Regulating Fluid Intake for Somebody with Advanced CKD

Individuals with acute CKD may need to restrict the amount they drink because damaged kidneys can't expel excess liquid. The liquid develops in the body and strains the heart. Patients should inform their doctor about any swelling around the eyes or in the legs, arms, or stomach area.

Importance of Keeping Track of and Understanding Lab Reports for Somebody with Advanced CKD

Figuring out how to read and understand lab reports gives an individual a chance to see how various foods can influence the kidneys. A doctor should arrange for normal blood tests for individuals with CKD. Patients can approach their doctor for copies of their lab reports and ask to have them clarified, taking note of any outcomes out of the ordinary range. Individuals with CKD should talk with their doctor or dietitian about how they can make better food decisions (PDF, 178 KB). For instance, if a test shows that an individual with CKD has a high potassium level, that individual should focus on lessening potassium in the diet by limiting high-potassium foods.

Clinical Trials

The National Institutes of Digestive and Diabetes and Kidney Diseases (NIDDK) and different parts of the National Institutes of Health (NIH) direct and bolster investigation into numerous diseases and conditions.

Clinical preliminaries are an aspect of clinical research that focuses on approaches to avoid, diagnose, or treat diseases. Specialists also use clinical preliminaries to consider different aspects of care, for example, improving the personal satisfaction of individuals with chronic diseases.

CHAPTER 6
DIET AND KIDNEY DISEASE

Get Started Learning About Eating With Kidney Disease

If you have kidney disease, your primary care physician will probably instruct you to be increasingly mindful with respect to the protein, sodium, potassium, phosphorus, and calcium in your diet. If you are in the beginning stages of CKD, there might be hardly any limits on what you can eat. However, as CKD advances, you must be more cautious about what you put into your body. For instance, individuals with kidney disease who are on dialysis will have different dietary needs from somebody with Stage 2 or 3 kidney disease.

Remember that every patient's dietary needs are unique – they're based on the phase of your kidney disease, your other ailments, your prescriptions, your weight, and your general health. Talk to a registered dietitian who specializes in kidney disease. A dietitian can help you make the best food decisions depending on your lab tests and way of life.

Patients who want to assume responsibility for their diets will find it helpful to work with a dietitian. Dietitians will enable you to plan your dinner, recognize food that is good for your kidneys, and create individualized eating plans that address your particular concerns and make eating a pleasant and nutritious experience.

DIET AND DIALYSIS

Figure Out How to Eat Well on Dialysis

A meal plan can play a major role in your dialysis treatment. A few aspects of a dialysis diet will carry over from the previous phases of kidney disease (lower salt, potassium, and phosphorus). However, there are two key things to screen for once you start dialysis: proteins and liquids.

- *Proteins:* Dialysis patients lose protein during treatment, which means they have to restore it by including more protein in their dinners. Protein can help keep up blood protein levels and improve wellbeing. Many specialists suggest that you eat high-protein food (meat, fish, poultry, fresh pork, eggs, and so on) at each supper, or around 8-10 ounces of protein-rich foods consistently.

- *Fluids:* Limiting liquids will enable you to feel better. When you're on dialysis, you may have trouble urinating. Any additional liquid must be expelled by dialysis. Consuming an excessive amount of liquid may cause problems between dialysis sessions, which may bring about migraines; swelling in your face, hands, and feet (edema); difficulty breathing; hypertension/stroke; and heart issues (due to stressing your heart with an excessive amount of liquid).

Liquids are commonly restricted on a dialysis diet. However, the amount you should have every day may depend upon your health and the sort of dialysis you're on. Individuals on at-home peritoneal dialysis may have less liquid diets, while individuals on in-focus hemodialysis for the most part have more restrictions in terms of their liquid consumption. Talk to your primary care physician or dietitian about how to deal with your liquids and feel your best.

DIET AND KIDNEY TRANSPLANTS

Investigate How Your Diet Changes After Receiving a Transplant

After a kidney transplant, your diet will help maintain your health. Dealing with your diet might be easier than it was when you were combating kidney disease or on dialysis.

Use the following list to learn about the role that nourishment can play post-transplant, and discover answers to questions common among patients living with a new kidney.

Do I Need to Be on a Special Diet?

Your diet is important after a kidney transplant. It is essential to maintain a sound weight and exercise routinely. A sound, balanced diet will help counteract high glucose and weight gain and will keep you healthy.

After a kidney transplant, plan to follow a diet low in salt. A good diet includes an assortment of fresh vegetables, lean meats, low-fat dairy items, whole grains, and a lot of water.

Also, you may need to abstain from eating particular kinds of foods. Your doctor can help you identify foods to avoid – and why. Your dietitian can also help you to discover a diet that is perfect for you.

If you were on dialysis and had a kidney transplant, you may find that this diet is simpler to follow than the one you were on for your dialysis.

Will Any Medications Influence My Diet?

Certainly. Your diet will be influenced by the drugs you take to prevent rejection of your transplant. Such medications include:

- Steroids (prednisone)
- Cyclosporine (Sandimmune, Neoral, Gengraf)
- Tacrolimus (Prograf)
- Azathioprine (Imuran)
- Mycophenolate (CellCept)

This list will keep growing as new prescriptions are created. These medications may change the manner in which your body works in various ways.

Should I Eliminate Any Foods?

After your kidney transplant, you should take unique prescriptions, called "immunosuppressive medications" or "anti-rejection drugs." These medications help eliminate the risk of organ rejection. However, these medications also debilitate your body's capacity to battle disease. Essentially, these prescriptions make you more prone to illness caused by germs.

A few germs cause bacterial diseases. Some bacterial diseases can be acquired from food. You can help bring down your danger of contamination from food by:

- Handling foods safely, such as washing your hands after touching raw chicken or eggs.
- Being cautious when eating out.
- Avoiding certain 'high-risk foods because they are bound to have microbes that can cause contamination.

You may also need to take steroids, which can cause:

- Increased craving, causing undesirable weight gain
- Increased blood fat levels (cholesterol and triglycerides)

- Salt and liquid retention
- A breakdown in muscle and bone tissue

Because of undesirable weight gain, it's critical to make sound food decisions and stick to appropriate portions. It might be a great idea to avoid greasy foods and foods high in basic sugar. Check with your doctor before you exercise. You may need to work out three or four times each week for 20-30 minutes each time.

Will I Put on Weight?

Many individuals have cravings after they get a transplant, and they put on undesirable weight. Check yourself frequently. Avoid unhealthy foods like greasy foods, desserts, cakes, and foods rich in carbs or fat. You can also maintain or control your calories by eating:

- Raw vegetables and fruits
- Lean meat, cleaned poultry, and fish
- Non-fat dairy items
- Sugar-free beverages

Controlling your weight will lower your risk of having issues, for example, coronary illness, diabetes, and hypertension. If you put on undesirable weight, you should exercise more and follow a low-calorie diet. Ask your doctor to refer you to a dietitian to plan low-calorie dinners and snacks.

What About Triglyceride and Cholesterol Levels?

Fat (cholesterol or triglyceride) levels in your blood might be high. Elevated levels of cholesterol and triglyceride can cause coronary illness. There are many ways you can lower the fat and cholesterol in your blood.

What About Foods High in Starches?

You should know some significant realities about foods high in sugars:

- Carbohydrates originate from sugars and starches.
- They give fuel and energy to your body.
- When you take prescription steroids, it is difficult for your body to use additional starches. This can prompt high glucose levels and may cause diabetes

Do I Have to Follow a Low-Salt Diet?

Many people still need to restrict salt after they get a transplant, though this differs with every individual. Transplant prescriptions, particularly steroids, may make your body retain liquid, and salt exacerbates this issue.

Excess liquid in the body increases circulatory strain. Controlling circulatory strain is essential to the health of your transplant. Your primary care physician will choose the amount of sodium that is best for you.

What About Protein?

Protein is significant for the following reasons:

- It creates and fixes muscles and tissues.
- It promotes healing after your transplant.

Your protein consumption should be higher than typical just after your transplant, to help develop the muscle tissue that will be separated by the large portions of steroids. Afterward, you can lower your protein intake.

What About Potassium?

So long as your transplant is successful, you should have the option to consume ordinary amounts of potassium from your food. However, some transplant medications can build your blood level of potassium, while different prescriptions may diminish it.

Are Phosphorus and Calcium an Issue?

You may need to give close consideration to your calcium and phosphorus levels. If you have been sick for a while, particularly if you had kidney disease, your body likely is deficient in the amount of calcium and phosphorus required for sound bones. In the months after your transplant, your primary care physician will check for possible bone loss and talk with you about the ideal approach to keeping your bones as sound as possible.

Meanwhile, every adult needs around two servings per day from the dairy group (low-fat milk, cheese, and yogurt). Unless your primary care physician or dietitian has told you to avoid these foods, try to include them in your dinners. Your primary care physician may determine that you need more calcium and phosphorus than your diet provides and may instruct you to take a supplement. Don't make any changes without talking to your doctor, as this could cause issues with your transplant.

What If I Have Diabetes?

After a transplant, your new diet might be higher in protein and lower in sugars because of the impacts of steroids and different drugs. Work with your primary care physician and dietitian to keep your diet and glucose under control.

DEALING WITH YOUR DIET

Many individuals living with kidney disease feel that the renal diet is the most difficult aspect of treatment. Dealing with a renal diet can be trying for various reasons:

- There is no standard "kidney diet" – it changes after some time based upon kidney work.
- Many individuals need to follow at least two diets, for example, a diabetic diet or potentially a heart-healthy diet alongside a renal diet.

- The diet can be truly restrictive, particularly if you have food allergies or limitations.
- Many of the rules and recommendations for good dieting don't apply when you're following a renal diet. You may need to avoid certain fruits, vegetables, and whole grains.

The renal diet can also affect your personal satisfaction and your social activities:

- Grocery shopping and preparing renal-friendly suppers can seem to be all-day work.
- It can be hard to eat out and still control your sodium, potassium, phosphorous, and protein consumption.
- Friends and family may not know or comprehend what you can eat.
- You may miss some of your favorite foods.

CHAPTER 7
ACUTE KIDNEY FAILURE

What Is Acute Kidney Failure?

Acute kidney failure occurs when your kidneys lose the ability to remove excess salts, liquids, and waste materials from the blood. This disposal is kidneys' primary job. Body liquids can ascend to risky levels when kidneys lose their filtering capacity. The condition will also cause a buildup of electrolytes and waste material in your body, which can be dangerous.

Acute kidney failure can happen quickly, over a couple of hours. It can also develop over a couple of days or weeks. Individuals who are always sick and need constant care are at the highest risk of acute kidney failure.

Acute kidney failure can be dangerous and requires intense treatment. However, it might be reversible. If you're generally healthy, recovery is possible.

Causes of Acute Kidney Failure

Acute kidney failure can happen for different reasons. Among the most widely recognized reasons are:

- Acute cylindrical corruption (ATN)
- Severe or unexpected drying out

- Kidney damage from toxic substances or certain medications
- Autoimmune kidney diseases, for example, intense nephritic disorder and interstitial nephritis
- Urinary tract block

Diminished blood flow can harm your kidneys. The following conditions can prompt diminished blood flow to your kidneys:

- Low circulatory strain
- Burns
- Dehydration
- Hemorrhage
- Injury
- Septic stun
- Serious disease
- Surgery

Certain conditions can cause thickening inside your kidney's veins, which can prompt acute kidney failure. These conditions include:

- Hemolytic uremic disorder
- Idiopathic thrombocytopenic thrombotic purpura (ITTP)
- Malignant hypertension
- Transfusion response
- Scleroderma

A few conditions, for example, septicemia and intense pyelonephritis, can easily harm your kidneys.

Pregnancy can also cause inconveniences that plague the kidneys, including placenta previa and placenta unexpectedness.

What Are the Risk Factors for Acute Kidney Failure?

The odds of suffering from acute kidney failure increase if you are older or suffer from one of the following chronic medical issues:

- Kidney disease
- Liver disease
- Diabetes, particularly if it's uncontrolled
- High circulatory strain
- Heart failure
- Obesity

If you're sick or being treated in a clinic's emergency unit, you are at a very high risk for acute kidney failure. Undergoing heart or stomach surgery, or receiving a bone marrow transplant, can also increase your risk.

Symptoms of Acute Kidney Failure

The signs and symptoms of acute kidney failure include the following:

- Bloody stools
- Mouth odor
- Sluggish and slow movements
- Fluid retention
- Fatigue
- Pain around hips and ribs
- Hand tremor
- Bruising easily
- Changes in mental status or disposition, particularly in older adults
- Reduced appetite
- Decreased sensation, particularly in your hands or feet
- Prolonged bleeding
- Seizures
- Nausea
- Vomiting
- Metallic taste in the mouth
- High blood pressure

How to Diagnose Acute Kidney Failure

With an acute kidney failure, you may suffer from bloating. This is because you are retaining liquids.

Utilizing a stethoscope, your primary care physician may hear snapping in the lungs. These sounds can indicate liquid retention.

Tests may also reveal symptoms of acute kidney failure. These tests include:

- Blood urea nitrogen (BUN)
- Serum potassium
- Serum sodium
- Estimated glomerular filtration rate (eGFR)
- Urinalysis
- Creatinine freedom
- Serum creatinine

An ultrasound is the best strategy for diagnosing acute kidney failure. However, a stomach X-ray, stomach CT scan, and stomach MRI can help your doctor decide whether there's a blockage in your urinary tract.

Certain blood tests may also uncover basic reasons for acute kidney failure.

Treatment for Acute Kidney Failure

Your treatment will rely upon the reason for your acute kidney failure. The objective is to reestablish ordinary kidney function. Preventing liquid retention while your kidneys recover is significant. In most cases, a kidney doctor called a "nephrologist" makes an assessment.

- **Diet**

Your primary care physician will limit your diet and the amount of fluids you can eat and drink. This will lessen the development of poisons that the kidneys would typically dispose of. A diet high in sugars and low in protein, salt, and potassium is normally prescribed.

- **Drugs**

Your primary care physician may prescribe anti-microbials to treat or prevent any diseases that happen concurrently. Diuretics may enable your kidneys to dispose of liquid. Calcium and insulin can help you avoid hazardous increases in your blood potassium levels.

- **Dialysis**

You may require dialysis. This procedure involves redirecting blood out of your body and into a machine that filters out waste. The clean blood then re-enters your body. If your potassium levels are perilously high, dialysis can save your life.

Dialysis is essential if there are changes in your psychological status or if you quit urinating. You may also require dialysis if you have pericarditis or heart disease. Dialysis can help remove nitrogen waste products from your body.

Complications of Acute Kidney Failure

Complications include the following:

- High blood pressure
- Kidney failure
- Heart damage
- Renal failure
- Nervous system damage

Preventing Acute Kidney Failure

Treating and preventing ailments that can prompt acute kidney failure is the best way to avoid the disease. As per the Mayo Clinic, following a lifestyle that includes regular physical movement and a reasonable diet can prevent kidney failure. Work with your primary care physician to monitor existing ailments that could prompt acute kidney failure.

What is the long-term viewpoint?

Acute kidney failure can be a hazardous ailment. There's a more serious risk of death if kidney failure is brought about by extreme contamination, injury, or a medical procedure.

The following can also increase the risk of death:

- Advanced age
- Lung disease

- Blood loss
- Recent stroke
- Kidney failure

With adequate treatment, your odds of recovery are great. Ask your primary care physician about what you can do to heal quicker.

PHASES OF KIDNEY DISEASE

It's important to know the five phases of kidney disease and the individual Glomerular Filtration Rate (GFR) values. A GFR blood test shows how well your kidneys are filtering and their general capacity. A higher GFR means your kidneys are working better, while a lower GFR indicates kidney decay.

Kidney Failure Abbreviations:

CKD: Chronic Kidney Disease

GFR: Glomerular Filtration Rate

BUN: Blood Urea Nitrogen

At stages 1–2: Symptoms of kidney disease are not clear

- Diet changes include limiting sodium to <2000 mg or as determined by your doctor.

- Medication, for example, ACE (angiotensin changing over catalyst) inhibitors and ARBs (angiotensin receptor blockers), are prescribed to help moderate renal decrease
- Patients on ACE inhibitors can experience expanded potassium levels and may need to restrict potassium in the diet if their doctors recommend it.
- Ingestion of fruits, veggies, and whole grains is encouraged.
- Control of cholesterol, glucose, and circulatory strain.
- Exercise/remaining active is prescribed to keep up an ordinary weight (BMI < 25 for adults).
- No smoking.
- Regular checkups to screen GFR and urine protein.

At stage 3:

At this stage, manifestations of kidney disease may be obvious. These may include liquid retention and exhaustion.

- Finding a nephrologist is necessary at this stage. Meeting with a dietician is also suggested. You can normally find one through your nephrologist's office.

- A dietician can work with your individual needs in counsel with your nephrologist to assess your protein consumption, phosphorus, potassium, uric acid, and hemoglobin (iron) levels.
- You may need to limit your phosphorus consumption depending upon your lab results. Maintaining all the treatment proposals from stages 1–2 is vital.
- Medication, for example, ACE (angiotensin changing over catalyst) inhibitors and ARBs (angiotensin receptor blockers), are prescribed to help moderate renal decay.

At stage 4:

In addition to the previously mentioned indications of kidney disease, patients with stage 4 CKD can encounter diminished hunger and a foul, metallic taste in their mouths or awful breath due to an overabundance of urea in the blood (BUN).

- At this stage, dialysis or potentially kidney transplantation will probably be required sooner rather than later. Your nephrologist will survey the kinds of dialysis and alternatives for transplant with you.
- Patients may end up weak during stage 4 as their red platelet count drops.

- Phosphorus might be restricted in your diet or you may need to take phosphorus "fasteners" – medications that affix to phosphorus in your stomach so it can't be consumed by your circulatory system.
- You may need to limit potassium in stage 4 CKD. However, talk with your primary care physician about your particular needs.

At stage 5:

Loss of hunger and restricted urine yield are basic during this. Patients may experience tingling because of high phosphorus levels in the blood.

- The medicines for stage 5 are hemodialysis, peritoneal dialysis, or kidney transplantation.
- Potassium consumption is intently checked and might be limited alongside liquid consumption.
- For patients who are on dialysis, a nephrology nutrient is frequently prescribed to compensate for water-soluble nutrients lost during dialysis. Talk with your doctor about whether nutrients or supplements are right for you.

CHAPTER 8
RENAL DIET FREQUENTLY
ASKED QUESTIONS

I have stage 3 CKD. What can I do to slow the progression of my kidney disease?

There are numerous approaches to help delay the progression of kidney disease, particularly if you are diagnosed in the early stages.

Listed below are a few hints that can help you protect your kidneys:

- *Eat healthily:* I recommend that you follow a balanced, adjusted diet that is limited in sodium. A decent method of restricting sodium is to avoid processed foods, (for example, quick foods, canned foods, packaged foods, and frozen foods). I also suggest that you avoid excessive protein (see FAQ 'how much protein do I need each day?'). Also, replacing some animal-based protein with vegetable protein may help moderate the advance of CKD. Avoiding high-phosphate foods (like colas, processed cheeses, and prepared meats) may also help safeguard your kidneys.

- *Monitor your blood pressure:* Research has demonstrated that great blood pressure can help moderate the advancement of kidney disease.
- *Stay active:* Make physical movement a habit. Thirty minutes of moderate physical activity every day is suggested.
- *Maintain a healthy weight:* Being overweight increases your risk for diabetes and hypertension, which are significant risk factors for kidney disease.
- *Stay hydrated:* Drink water rather than calorie-rich beverages.
- *If you take alcohol, consume it in moderation:* Limit your alcohol consumption to two standard beverages per day for men, and one per day for women (see FAQ 'how much liquor is alright for kidney patients?').
- *If you have diabetes:* Always monitor and maintain great blood glucose.
- *Do not smoke:* Smoking is a risk factor for the advancement of kidney disease.
- *Take drugs* as prescribed by your physician.
- *Get regular checkups* with your physician.
- *Maintain a positive 'healthy' attitude* and accomplish things that will help you unwind and decrease stress.

Keep in mind it is never too late to roll out positive improvements to your way of life. Eating well and keeping active can improve your long-term and help your kidneys function well.

How much protein do I need every day?

Because protein needs can depend on your drugs, other illness, or your general health status, it is ideal to talk with a renal dietitian about the amount of protein that will enable you to remain healthy. If you have stage 1-4 kidney disease, you should go for 0.8 grams of protein per kilogram of body weight. This adds up to around one or two servings of low-phosphorus meat and alternatives, each about the size of a deck of cards, every day. If you are on dialysis, you will lose some protein during the filtration process, so you should go for 1.1-1.3 grams of protein per kilogram every day. This adds up to two or three servings of low-phosphorus meat and alternatives – again, each about the size of a deck of cards.

Being physically active doesn't necessary mean that you need more protein. However, extra protein is suggested for pregnant or lactating women.

How can I meet my protein needs when I'm not hungry, or if I don't like meat?

Animal protein foods like beef, sheep, pork, poultry, and fish are exceptionally rich in protein. Eating these protein-rich foods makes it easier to meet your dietary protein needs.

However, this meat should be consumed in limited quantities. Eat small amounts of protein more frequently or add meat to other dishes —for example, soups, salads, pastas, sandwiches, and so on. Individuals who don't like red meat or poultry may like fish. Fish is a phenomenal source of protein. Eggs and low-phosphorus cheese (for example, softer cheeses like brie, camembert, and goat, curds) can also help address protein issues. It is critical to talk with your dietitian to determine how much meat, egg, and cheese is suitable for you.

Some people don't eat meat for various reasons, such as taste aversions and religious beliefs. These individuals might be able to consume more dairy products, tofu, or vegetables to meet their protein needs. However, dairy items and vegetables cause an increase in blood phosphorus levels. Talk to your dietitian about your blood levels and food consumption.

At the point when standard foods are not adequate to address protein issues, you might need to use protein supplements. Supplements may include protein powders that are blended into different foods or high-protein beverages. Talk to your dietitian before using protein supplements and get information about kidney-accommodating high-protein foods that may enable you to meet your protein needs.

What amount of liquor is acceptable for individuals with kidney disease?

Moderate liquor use might be alright. However, it's ideal to talk about this with your doctor. Consuming too much alcohol can lead to hypertension, high blood triglyceride levels, or damage to the pancreas or liver. It might also clash with your prescriptions. Furthermore, liquor may make your blood pressure or glucose level increasingly hard to control, and can prompt weight gain.

If you are drinking liquor, drink only one or two standard beverages daily – 14 beverages per week for men and 10 beverages per week for women.

Standard drinks are:

- 355-milliliter can of 5% beer
- 146-milliliter glass of 10-12% wine
- 44 milliliters of 40% spirit or hard alcohol

Special considerations:

- Because alcohol adds liquid to the body, individuals with CKD, and particularly those on dialysis, are encouraged to restrict their liquid consumption.
- Certain mixed drinks are higher in potassium or phosphorus than others:
  - Red wine contains more potassium than white wine.

- Beer is a critical source of potassium and phosphorus.
- Spirits – for example, vodka, rum, and gin – contain almost no potassium or phosphorus.
- Mixes served with liquor might be high in potassium as well as phosphorus. (For instance, orange juice is high in potassium and colas are regularly high in potassium as well as phosphorus.)

Do all individuals with kidney disease need to follow a fluid restriction diet?

Your primary care physician might suggest a liquid diet. However, this is not always necessary, so be sure to ask your doctor.

How can I tell if a food is high or low in potassium based on the nutrition facts?

Have you ever asked why a few items list potassium in the nutrition facts table, while others don't? Potassium isn't always recorded in the nutrition facts table because it isn't one of the 13 core supplements that are compulsory to list. Brands that list potassium may do so because the manufacturer has decreased the amount of sodium in the product by including potassium salts, or because the manufacturer wants to show that the product is a good source of potassium. The fact one item lists potassium and a comparable item doesn't is not an indication that the comparable item contains zero potassium. Practically all foods contain potassium. For instance, one brand of apple juice may list 200 mg of potassium in three-quarters of a cup of juice, while another brand of apple juice may not list potassium in the nutrition facts table. Likely, the two brands of apple juice contain around 200 mg of potassium per three-quarters of a cup, but the laws don't require that potassium content be recorded.

If a nutrition facts table contains potassium, what do the numbers mean? The following rules might be valuable in helping you determine whether a particular food has a lot, or little, potassium (consistently check with your renal dietitian for individual rules):

- Very low potassium: under 40 mg per serving (1 %)
- Low potassium: under 100 mg per serving (3%)
- Medium potassium: 100-250 mg per serving (3-7%)
- High potassium: 250-500 mg per serving (7-14%)
- Very high potassium: over 500 mg per serving (>14%)

Do I have to take nutrient and mineral supplements?

Nutrients are found in the foods we eat and have numerous functions in the human body. Eating an assortment of foods is the most ideal approach to get the majority of your nutrients. However, individuals with chronic kidney disease (CKD) may not get enough of certain nutrients as a result of their diets, or due to nutrient loss during dialysis. CKD patients, particularly those on dialysis, may require additional water-dissolvable nutrients like B vitamins. A few nutrients and minerals must be restricted or avoided because their levels can increase in the body as the kidneys quit working. These are the fat-soluble nutrients (like An, E, and K) and minerals such as potassium and phosphorus. They shouldn't be augmented except if requested by your primary care physician. An everyday nutrient supplement explicitly intended for kidney patients is frequently prescribed. If your doctor has not prescribed a nutrient supplement, ask whether you would benefit from one. Use only the nutrient supplement prescribed by your doctor.

I have kidney disease and I'm taking a natural supplement. Is this safe?

Like certain nutrients, some natural supplements can be unsafe to individuals with kidney disease. Talk with your primary care physician, dietitian, or renal drug specialist if you are taking any natural arrangements. Your doctor can tell you which supplements might be of concern.

Can I consume artificial sweeteners?

Yes, artificial sweeteners are safe for use by chronic kidney disease patients.

However, care should to be taken to ensure that one purchases sugars that have been approved by the health authorities.

Following are the various kinds of sugars that have been prescribed for use in Canada (for instance):

- *Aspartame* is advertised under the brand names Equal™ and NutraSweet. It's used in soda pop, yogurt, and snacks, and as a tabletop sugar. It contains phenylalanine, so individuals with phenylketonuria (PKU) must stay away from aspartame.
- *Sucralose* is sold under the brand name Splenda. It is broadly used in soda pop, treats, prepared foods, and frozen sweets and frozen yogurt. It is also used for home cooking.
- *Acesulfame* potassium isn't used as a tabletop sugar. It's used only by food makers as an element for improving soda pop and treats.
- *Sugar alcohols* (sorbitol, mannitol, maltitol, xylitol) can't be purchased as table sugars. They are used by food makers in foods and refreshments such as snacks, frozen sweets, and frozen yogurt. Sugar alcohols are "false" sugar substitutes –

they contain limited quantities of calories which may influence blood glucose (sugar) levels. Huge sums (in excess of 10 grams/day) can cause diarrhea, gas, and bloating.

- *Saccharin* is promoted as the tabletop sugar Hermesetas. It must be purchased at drug stores in Canada. If you are pregnant, check with your doctor before using saccharin.
- *Stevia* leaf and the concentrate of stevia leaves are approved for use in certain health products, Refined stevia extract, otherwise called "steviol glycoside", is used as a tabletop sugar and is added to certain foods, like snacks, gum, etc.

For pregnant and breastfeeding women

If you are pregnant or breastfeeding, sugar substitutes, including aspartame, acesulfame potassium, sucralose, and sugar alcohols are viewed as safe. However, don't substitute artificial sweeteners for the nutrient-rich foods you require for a healthy pregnancy.

For children and infants

It is suggested that babies and kids stay away from artificial sweeteners.

What should I do if I have no appetite?

Loss of appetite is a typical issue when the kidneys cannot remove waste from the blood. You need enough protein and calories to stay healthy and avoid muscle loss.

If you have a poor appetite:

- Eat small dinners and fatty snacks throughout the day (every two to three hours).
- Eat your biggest meal when your cravings are at their highest. If you're not hungry at night, have your biggest meal at breakfast or lunch.
- Carry snacks with you if you will be away from home during the day. Examples include cheese and crackers, or a sandwich.
- Schedule suppers and snacks.
- Experiment with various foods; for example, try cold foods rather than a hot meal.
- Make a list of simple or most-loved dinners and take a look at it when you don't know what to eat.
- Try going for a walk or getting some fresh air. This may make you hungry.
- Ask your dietitian about a kidney-accommodating fluid supplement.
- Make each piece count. Include additional protein and calories:
  - Add margarine to rice, noodles, saltines, vegetables, and bread.

- Use nectar, jam, margarine, or cream cheese on toast, bread, and saltines.
- Mix cooked ground beef, chicken, or turkey into soups, pasta, or rice.
- Add cheese to vegetables, salads, etc.
- Add a hard-boiled egg or fish to your salad.
- Spread peanut butter on crackers or bread.
- Add tofu to soups, stews, etc.
- Use "good" fats generously. Try dunking bread in olive oil.
- Sauté foods in canola or olive oil.
- Add low-salt dressings to salads and vegetables.
- Drink beverages that contain calories.
- Avoid "light" or "diet" foods

I had a kidney transplant. What kind of diet do I have to follow?

Each transplant is unique and as you progress, your blood work will help your primary care physician and renal dietitian determine what foods to include in your diet. Your protein requirements are generally higher after a transplant so as to promote healing and as a result of the steroids you will be taking to prevent organ rejection. Your blood sugar may also be higher due to the steroids, particularly if you have diabetes. Your primary care physician can help you manage your blood sugars. The steroid prescriptions will also increase your calcium requirements, so you should concentrate on consuming calcium-rich foods to keep your bones healthy. Continue following a low-sodium diet unless your doctor indicates otherwise.

Frequently, a higher consumption of whole grains, wheat, nuts and seeds, beans, and lentils is prescribed to guarantee that you get sufficient amounts of minerals like phosphorus and magnesium. Finally, you might experience weight gain post-transplant because you will have a bigger appetite. Therefore, you will want to plan accordingly. Ask your doctor for a referral to a renal dietitian, who can give you information about which foods to include in your diet.

CHAPTER 9
RENAL DIET RECIPES AND
MENU CHOICES

MENU CHOICES

Salads and Appetizers

- Look for new, basic options to avoid excessive salt or liquid.
- Ask which vegetables are in the salad if the menu doesn't indicate this fact.

Better Choices: Chef salad, crab cakes, garlic bread without cheese, seared zucchini, or onion rings

Courses

- Watch your portions; try to assess the amount you typically would eat at home. Request a container to take the additional home.
- Avoid blended dishes or meals that are frequently higher in salt and phosphorus.
- Remove the skin from poultry to help reduce the salt content.

Better Choices: barbecued or seared steaks, prime rib, cheeseburger without cheese, fajitas, pan-fried (flame-broiled or simmered) options, and sandwiches

Side Dishes

- Go for starches and vegetables that are lower in potassium if you are on a potassium restriction.
- Save your vegetable options during the day to give you more alternatives when you are eating out.
- Ask for a substitute if necessary.

Better Choices: rice, noodles, green beans, blended vegetables

Pastries

- Avoid pastries made with chocolate, cream cheese, frozen yogurt, or nuts, which will be higher in potassium and phosphorus – or share with a companion.
- Low-potassium fruits are a good choice, particularly if you have diabetes.

Better Choices: low-potassium natural products, organic ice products, sorbet, apple, blueberry, lemon meringue pies, strawberry shortcake.

RECIPES

BANNOCK

Ingredients:

- 1½ cups all-purpose flour
- 2 teaspoons powdered milk
- 2 tablespoons vegetable oil
- ½ cup water

Preparation:

- Preheat stove to 400°F.
- Mix flour and powdered milk. Blend in oil until the mixture looks brittle. Add water. Mix well. Pour in container.
- Bake for 15 minutes.

Nutritional Information:

Makes 8 servings

1 serving = 1 starch and 1 fat

(16 grams carbohydrates, 3 grams fat).

BEEF AND BARLEY STEW

Ingredients:

- 1 cup uncooked pearl barley
- 1 pound lean hamburger stew meat, cut into 1½-inch shapes
- 2 tablespoons flour
- 2 tablespoons oil
- ½ cup diced onion
- 1 large stalk celery, cut
- 1 clove garlic, minced
- 2 carrots, cut ¼ inch thick
- 2 straight leaves
- 1 teaspoon Mrs. Run onion herb flavoring

Preparation:

1. Soak barley in water for 60 minutes.
2. Put flour, black pepper, and stew meat in a plastic container.
3. Shake to coat stew meat with flour.
4. Warm oil in large 4-quart pot and darken stew meat. Remove meat from cooking pot. Sauté onion, celery, and garlic in meat drippings for 2 minutes.
5. Add 2 quarts of water and heat to point of boiling. Return meat to pot. Add straight leaves and salt. Return to a simmer.

6. Drain and rinse grains. Add to pot. Spread and cook for 60 minutes. Mix at regular intervals.

7. After 1 hour, add carrots and Mrs. Run flavoring. Stew for one more hour. Add extra water if necessary.

Nutritional Information:

6 servings

1¼ cup (3 meat and alternate, 1 bread and starch, 1 medium vegetable)

BLUEBERRY LEMON MUFFINS

Ingredients:

- 1 cup all-purpose flour
- ¾ cup whole-wheat flour
- ½ cup granulated sugar
- 2 teaspoons baking powder
- ½ teaspoon baking soda
- 1 tablespoon ground lemon or orange strip
- 1 ½ cups Coffee Rich®
- 2 egg whites
- 1 cup fresh or frozen unsweetened blueberries

Preparation:

- Preheat stove to 375°F.
- In a large bowl, mix flours with sugar, baking powder, baking soda, and lemon strip until well-blended.
- Whisk Coffee Rich with margarine and egg whites in a medium bowl until mixed.
- Mix Coffee Rich blend into flour blend until mixed.
- Add blueberries.
- Spoon into lightly greased, non-stick, or paper-lined biscuit tins.

- Heat for 20-22 minutes, until slightly golden on top and a toothpick embedded in the muffins comes out clean.
- Makes 12 muffins.

Nutritional Information:

1 serving = 1 biscuit (1 starch and ½ low potassium natural product)

CRANBERRY SPARERIBS

Ingredients:

- 3 pounds spareribs
- ¼ cup (50 ml) dark-colored sugar
- 3 tablespoons (45 ml) flour
- ¼ teaspoon (1 ml) dry mustard
- ¼ teaspoon (1 ml) grounded cloves
- 14-ounce can (355ml) cranberry sauce
- 2 tablespoons (30 ml) vinegar
- 1 tablespoon lemon juice
- 2 cups water

Preparation:

- Place ribs on grill rack. Cook until dark-colored. Turn and cook on other side.
- Pour off drippings and wash ribs under warm water. Place ribs in goulash dish.
- Blend sugar, flour, mustard, and cloves in pot. Add remaining ingredients.
- Cook and mix over medium heat until somewhat thick.
- Pour sauce over ribs. Spread. Cook at 350°F for 60 minutes. Uncover for last 15-20 minutes.

Nutritional Information:

Serves: 6

(protein, 1 starch, 2½ fruits and vegetables, 2 fats)

GRILLED FISH IN FOIL

Ingredients:

- 1 pound fish filets, fresh or frozen (and defrosted)
- 2 tablespoons margarine
- Mrs. Dash® (or McCormick's No Salt Added®)

Pepper:

- 1 medium onion, daintily cut
- 1 lemon, cut into wedges

Preparation:

- Preheat open-air flame broil for medium heat.
- On 4 large buttered squares of aluminum foil, place equivalent amounts of fish (about 3 ounces per foil parcel).
- Sprinkle each serving of fish with Mrs. Dash (season well) and pepper.
- Top each with onion and lemon wedge. (Crush lemon wedge over fish filet first.)
- Firmly wrap filets in foil (to prevent spilling) and place on flame broil.
- Barbecue 5-7 minutes on each side or until fish drops from fork.

Note: Thick fish filets may take more time to cook.

Nutritional Information:

Makes 4 servings

Supplements per 1 foil bundle: 3 meat servings

GRILLED CORN ON THE COB

Ingredients:

- 4 cobs of corn with husks
- Margarine
- Pepper to taste
- 4 squares of aluminum foil, large enough to wrap individual cobs

Preparation:

- Preheat flame broil to 400°F.
- Strip corn husks and remove silk (the hair on the corn). Add margarine and pepper to each cob of corn.
- Close husks. Wrap each ear of corn firmly in aluminum foil. Ensure edges are fixed firmly to avoid spilling. Add to barbecue.
- Cook around 25 to 30 minutes until corn is soft.

Nutritional Information:

Makes 4 servings

Supplements per 1 cob of corn: 2 medium vegetable

Be cautious; the corn will be extremely hot.

HERBED CHICKEN

Ingredients:

- 4 chicken breasts (fresh)
- 2 tablespoons herbed prepared flour (see recipe below)
- 2 tablespoons margarine
- ½ cup low-sodium chicken stock

Preparation:

- Dredge chicken in prepared flour.
- Melt margarine. Cook chicken until caramelized, around 3-5 minutes on each side.
- Pour chicken stock and cook, blending until softly thickened. Lessen heat to medium and cook, secured, for 3-4 minutes on each side or until chicken is no longer pink.

For stove:

- Put the chicken in a big dish and sprinkle with prepared flour.
- Pour ½ cup water onto chicken and cook at 400°F for about 45 minutes or until chicken is no longer pink.

Makes: 4 servings

Herbed-Seasoned Flour:

Combine: ½ cup flour, 1 teaspoon oregano, 2 teaspoons thyme, 2 teaspoons basil, 1 teaspoon tarragon, 1 teaspoon paprika, and ½ teaspoon ground black pepper.

LINGUINE WITH GARLIC AND SHRIMP

Ingredients:

- 2½ quarts water
- ¾ pound linguine pasta, uncooked
- 2 tablespoons olive oil
- ½ pound shrimp, peeled and cleaned
- 1 cup leaf parsley
- 1 tablespoon lemon juice
- Black pepper to taste

Preparation:

- Boil water in large pot. Add pasta and cook for 10 minutes or until soft.
- While cooking pasta, separate garlic cloves, leaving on skin. Heat cloves in skillet over medium heat, mixing every now and then.
- The garlic is ready when it softens. The skin will be easy to remove. Remove garlic from skillet and strip off skin. Warm olive oil in griddle and return peeled garlic to skillet.
- Cook garlic until golden. (Cloves can be sliced down the middle or left whole.) Add parsley and shrimp and cook 1 to 2 minutes, until shrimp turns pink. Drain pasta and reserve 1 cup fluid.
- Add pasta to container with shrimp and garlic. Combine all ingredients and add reserved cup

fluid. Add lemon juice and black pepper. Blend and serve.

Nutritional Information:

Servings: 4

Serving size: 2 cups

Supplements per serving: 3 meat (approx. 15½ large shrimp); 4 bread/starch; 1 vegetable, low potassium

LOW PHOSPHORUS PANCAKES

Ingredients:

- ½ cup rice or coffee-rich milk substitute
- ½ cup flour
- 1 egg
- 1 teaspoon sugar or Splenda
- 1 tablespoon vegetable oil

Preparation:

- Blend all ingredients well.
- Soften enough non-hydrogenated margarine to cover base of the skillet, which should be very hot. Pour about ¼ cup of hotcake blend in skillet and tip slightly every which way so the batter covers the base.
- Cook for around one minute, or until edges begin to turn golden. At that point, turn with a spatula to cook opposite side.
- Repeat for every pancake.

Makes 4 pancakes.

1 pancake = 1 serving breads and starch

ONION SMOTHERED STEAK

Ingredients:

- ¼ cup flour
- ⅛ teaspoon pepper
- ½ pound round steak, ¾-inch thick
- 2 tablespoons oil
- 1 cup water
- 1 tablespoon vinegar
- 1 clove garlic, minced
- 1 sound leaf
- ¼ teaspoon dried thyme
- 3 medium sliced onions

Preparation:

- Cut steak into 8 equal servings. Add flour and pepper and pound into meat.
- Heat oil in skillet and cook meat on both sides. Remove from skillet and put in a safe spot.
- Mix water, vinegar, garlic, leaf, and thyme in skillet. Heat to point of boiling.
- Add meat to this blend and spread with cut onions. Stew for one hour.

Serving: 8 – 2 oz meat for each serving.

RENAL AND RENAL DIABETIC EXCHANGES RECIPES

PORK SOUVLAKI

Ingredients:

- 1 pound pork, cut in 1-inch pieces
- ¼ cup oil
- 3 tablespoons lemon juice
- 1 teaspoon oregano, ground
- ¼ teaspoon black pepper
- 1 large garlic clove, minced

Preparation:

- Cut off excess from pork and cut in blocks. Put in a safe spot.
- In a bowl, add remaining ingredients and blend well. Add pork to marinade blend in bowl and let sit for 1-4 hours.
- Pan-fry pork in skillet over medium heat for 7-10 minutes until cooked.
- Put pork on sticks and flame-broil over medium heat on grill until done, turning once during cooking.

POTASSIUM-FRIENDLY HASH BROWNS

Ingredients:

- 2 cups potassium-friendly pureed potatoes
- 1 egg, beaten
- 1 onion, minced
- ⅛ teaspoon pepper
- 2-3 tablespoons olive oil

Preparation:

- Combine pureed potatoes, beaten egg, and onion in a medium bowl and add pepper.
- Over medium heat, heat olive oil in a medium-size non-stick skillet.
- Add about ¼ cup of potato blend into the skillet, tapping it into 4-inch circles that are ½ inch thick.
- Cook until base is sautéed and fresh, around 3-4 minutes.
- Carefully turn over patty and cook other side until it is dark-colored and fresh, about 3-4 minutes.

POTASSIUM-FRIENDLY MASHED POTATOES

Ingredients:

- Large cooking pot or dish of water

- 2 cups heating potatoes (2 large potatoes)

- ¼ cup polyunsaturated margarine

- ¼ mug Coffee Rich or Original Rice Dream

Preparation:

- Strip and cut potatoes into little pieces. Add to large pot of water.
- Bring gradually to boil; boil for 10 minutes. Remove water.
- Add cold water and gradually bring to a boil. Cook until done.
- Remove water. Pound potatoes with potato masher until soft.
- Gradually add margarine and Coffee Rich or Original Rice Dream until velvety.

POTATO SALAD

Ingredients:

- 2 cups diced potato (2 large potatoes)
- 3 tablespoons finely sliced celery
- 3 tablespoons finely sliced onion
- 3 tablespoons finely sliced green pepper
- 2 sliced hard-boiled eggs
- ¼ cup mayonnaise
- 2 teaspoons vinegar
- ⅛ teaspoon dry mustard
- ⅛ teaspoon dried parsley
- ⅛ teaspoon paprika
- 1 squeeze pepper
- 1 squeeze garlic powder

Preparation:

- Boil potatoes.
- Drain and refrigerate.
- Add vegetables and eggs to potatoes.
- In a different bowl, combine mayonnaise, vinegar, dry mustard, parsley, paprika, pepper, and garlic powder.
- Pour prepared mayonnaise over cooled potato blend.
- Stir softly to blend.
- Garnish with paprika and dried parsley.

Double-Boil Method:

- Peel and cut potatoes into little pieces. Add to large pot of water.
- Bring gradually to a boil; boil for 10 minutes. Remove water.
- Cover with cold water. Bring gradually to boil. Cook until done.
- Remove water.

QUICK CANNED PEAR DESSERT

Ingredients:

- 1/3 cup unsifted flour
- ¼ cup sugar
- ¼ cup unsalted butter or margarine
- 3 cups canned pears
- 2 tablespoons lemon juice
- ¼ cup sherry
- ¼ teaspoon nutmeg

Preparation:

- Preheat stove to 350°F.
- Mix flour with sugar in a medium bowl.
- With two blades or cake blender, cut margarine or spread and flour until blend is brittle.
- Put in a safe spot.
- Drain canned pears. Place cut pears into well-greased 9-inch pie plate.
- Sprinkle with lemon juice, sherry, and nutmeg.
- Sprinkle flour blend over top.
- Prepare in hot stove for 15 minutes or until sautéed

Makes 5 servings; 1 serving = ½ cup (1 starch and 1 low potassium natural product, 2 fat)

RENAL-FRIENDLY BRAN MUFFINS

Preheat broiler to 400°F and lightly grease biscuit tins.

Blend:

- ¼ cup oil
- 1 egg
- 1 teaspoon vanilla
- 1/3 cup nectar
- 1 cup fruit purée or squashed pineapple, drained

Add:

- 1 cup white flour
- 1 cup wheat grain
- ½ teaspoon baking soda
- ¼ teaspoon cream of tartar

Combine, spoon into biscuit tins, and heat right away. The cream of tartar and baking soda will rise once, so don't delay in getting the biscuits into the broiler. Heat for 15-20 minutes.

Makes 12 biscuits

1 biscuit = 1 starch, 1 low potassium

ROASTED RED PEPPER PIZZA

Ingredients:
Pizza:

- 1 Greek-style pita
- 2 tablespoons broiled red pepper sauce
- ¼ cup cooked ground hamburger
- 1 tablespoon green pepper, diced
- 1 tablespoon onion, diced
- 2 tablespoons brie, diced
- 2 tablespoons mozzarella, ground

Simmered Red Pepper Sauce:

- 1 whole red pepper, simmered
- 1-2 cloves garlic
- Black pepper
- 1 teaspoon olive oil

Preparation:

Pizza: Preheat broiler to 350°F. Place pita on preparing sheet and spread broiled red pepper sauce on it. Top with hamburger, green peppers, onion, and cheeses. Prepare for 10 minutes or until cheddar has softened and pizza is warmed through

Simmered Red Pepper Sauce: Heat pepper in oven or on BBQ until skin turns dark. Allow pepper to chill, then strip off skin. Puree peppers, garlic, black pepper, and olive oil in a food processor or blender until smooth.

Makes 1 serving: 2 starch, 3 protein, 1 low potassium vegetable

SALAD DRESSINGS and MARINADES

These dressings can also be used as a marinade for fish, poultry, and meat.

Essential Dressing

- ¼ cup red wine vinegar
- ¼ teaspoon garlic powder
- ¼ teaspoon dry mustard
- ½ teaspoon sugar
- ¼ cup water
- ¼ teaspoon ground black pepper
- 2 tablespoon fresh lemon juice
- 1 cup corn or olive oil

(Makes 1-1½ cups)

Mix all ingredients and place in a container with a tight-fitting cover. Shake well. Store, covered, in the icebox/refrigerator.

Curry Dressing

- 1 teaspoon curry powder
- ⅛ teaspoon ground ginger
- 1 – 1½ cups Basic Dressing

Add curry powder and ginger to the Basic Dressing and blend.

Italian Dressing

- 2 teaspoons dried oregano
- 1 teaspoon dried basil
- 1 teaspoon dried tarragon
- ½ teaspoon sugar
- 1 – 1½ cups Basic Dressing

Add oregano, basil, tarragon, and sugar to Basic Dressing and blend completely. Cover and store in refrigerator.

TURKEY and PASTA SALAD

Ingredients:

- 16 ounces unsalted, cooked turkey breast, cubed
- 3 cups elbow, shell, or tie pasta
- ¼ cup sliced celery
- 2 tablespoons sliced red pepper
- 2 tablespoons sliced carrot
- 2 tablespoons finely sliced purple onion
- ⅛ teaspoon pepper
- ½ cup mayonnaise
- ½ teaspoon sugar
- 1 tablespoon lemon juice

Preparation:

- Blend turkey, pasta, celery, red pepper, carrot, and purple onion in bowl.
- In a different bowl, mix dressing. Mix pepper, mayonnaise, sugar, and lemon juice until smooth.
- Pour dressing over pasta and vegetables and blend until all covered.
- Chill and serve.

Serves: 5

Serving Size: 1 cup

Supplements per serving: 3 meat; 1½ starch; 1 vegetable

VEGETABLE OMELET

Ingredients:

- ¼ cup cut green pepper
- ½ cup cut onions
- 1/3 cup frozen blended vegetables, steamed
- 2 eggs
- 2 egg whites
- 1 tablespoon unsalted margarine
- 2 tablespoons water

Preparation:

- Sauté green pepper and onion in unsalted marga-rine in a small skillet.
- Beat egg and water; add to skillet and cook until done.
- Add cooked blended vegetables
- Put on plate

1 serving: 1 protein, 1 low potassium vegetable

RENAL DIET: VEGETARIAN RECIPES

CAULIFLOWER CHEESE

This recipe uses both milk and cheese, which may seem to indicate that it is high in phosphate and potassium. It creates a lot of cauliflower cheese to serve 4-6 individuals. Per serving, it contains 25g/1oz of cheese and 125ml/¼ of milk, which is within the allowances for those requiring limitations.

Ingredients:

- 1 large cauliflower (leaves cut off), broken into pieces
- 500 milliliters milk
- 4 tablespoons flour
- 50 grams (1¾ ounces) spread
- 100 grams (3½ ounces) solid cheddar, ground
- 2-3 tablespoons breadcrumbs, optional

Preparation:

- Bring large pot of water to boil. Add cauliflower and cook for 5 minutes. Remove a piece to test; it should be cooked. Drain cauliflower and pour into ovenproof dish.
- Heat broiler to 220°C/425°F/Gas 7.
- Set the pan back on the heat and add milk, flour, and margarine. Whisk quickly as spread melts

and blend boils. The flour will vanish and the sauce will start to thicken. Mix for 2 minutes while sauce boils and thickens. Lower the heat, mix in most of the cheddar, and pour over cauliflower. Scatter over the rest of cheddar and breadcrumbs.

- Put cauliflower cheese in broiler for 20 minutes.

Tip: Makes enough for 6 servings. Extra portions can be frozen.

PUMPKIN RISOTTO

This is a filling dish and while it contains butternut squash (a vegetable with moderate amounts of potassium), it is made with rice (as opposed to potatoes), which lowers the potassium content of the overall dish. The cheese used in this recipe is minimal, but you can also make it without cheese to further lower the phosphate and fat.

Ingredients:

- 570 ml (16 ounces) low-salt bouillon or chicken stock
- 1 small onion, sliced
- 12 fresh sage leaves, chopped finely
- 2 tablespoons olive oil
- 170 grams (6 ounces) Arborio (risotto) rice
- 250 grams (9 ounces) pumpkin or butternut squash, diced
- 50 grams (2 ounces) margarine
- Freshly ground black pepper
- Piece of fresh parmesan, or parmesan-style grinding cheese (optional)

Preparation:

- Heat the stock until boiling and after that stew over low heat. In a different pan, sauté the onion in the oil until soft yet not seared. Add the sliced sage and cook for a couple more minutes.

- Add the rice and blend well for a couple of minutes to cover the grains with oil. At that point, pour in 1/3 of the stock and bring to a gentle stew. Cook until almost all the stock is gone. Add the pumpkin or squash and a little more stock and keep on stewing gently until the stock is gone.

- Add the remaining stock a little at a time, until the pumpkin is soft and the rice is still somewhat firm. You may not require all the stock.

- Mix the spread into the risotto, and season well with salt and pepper.

PASTRY-LESS QUICHE

This is a flexible recipe in that you can replace any of the vegetables with any of your preferred ingredients – for instance, peas and dried mint or squash and sage instead of the peppers. This dish can also be eaten hot or cold, making it great for supper at home or had in a boxed lunch. Note that tomatoes and mushrooms are both high-potassium foods yet are okay when eaten in modest quantities.

Ingredients:

- 1 green pepper, diced
- 1 red pepper, diced
- 1 onion, chopped
- 8 medium mushrooms, cut
- 2 large or 3 medium tomatoes, cut
- 5 eggs
- 250 grams (9 ounces) fat-free regular curds
- 75 milliliters milk
- 50 grams (1¾ ounces) ground cheddar, or use a lower phosphate cheddar, for example, feta

Preparation:

- Delicately fry the prepared vegetables (aside from the tomatoes) using either a small amount of vegetable oil or a splash of oil. They should still be a little crunchy.

- Combine the 5 eggs, 250g non-fat regular curds and the milk. This won't look pretty but stay with it.
- Spread the sliced vegetables out in a stove in a baking pan.
- Put the cut tomatoes over the top and sprinkle with the cheddar
- Bake in the stove at 190°C (170°C Fan)/375°F/Gas 5, for around 30-45 minutes, or until the quiche is set and dark-colored.

THE VERSATILE MINCE SECTION

This section is devoted to the flexibility of mince, and includes a wide range of recipes: pork, sheep, chicken, turkey, and veggie lover mince. You can choose which mince you would like to use for every one of these recipes. If you are attempting to shed pounds, you might want to choose lean or extra-lean meat, chicken, or turkey. Also, you may wish to try vegan mince, as this is also normally low-fat and a decent source of protein.

KIDNEY-FRIENDLY PASTY

These pasties are incredible served hot from the stove, though they are also great served cold in a boxed lunch. We suggest heating up the swede and carrot in this recipe, as this helps bring down the potassium content of these vegetables.

Ingredients:

- 250 grams (8 ounces) mince
- 1 medium onion, finely sliced
- 1 medium carrot, peeled and sliced
- ½ little swede or ¼ large one, peeled and chopped
- 2 teaspoons dried parsley
- 120 milliliters low-salt stock
- ½ teaspoon English mustard

- 500 grams (17 ounces) instant short-hull baked good
- 1 medium egg, softly whisked
- Pepper

Preparation:

- Pre-heat the broiler to 180°C (160°C Fan)/350°F.
- On the hob, heat up the sliced swede and carrot for 5-10 minutes or until somewhat soft. Then remove the water. (This helps bring down the potassium content of these vegetables.) Allow the vegetable to cool.
- In a different bowl, add the parsley, stock, onion, minced hamburger, and English mustard.
- Use a blade to cut the minced hamburger into little strands. Combine with your hands so the ingredients are spread equally all through the blend. Season with pepper.
- Add the cooled vegetables and gently mix with your mince blend.
- Take the mixture and roll it flat with a rolling pin to about 3mm thick. Press a saucer over it and create round slices. Place a portion of the filling on each circle.
- Brush a small amount of the egg around the edges of the pastry. Bring two edges of the pastry together to make a 'package' and crease the edges together.

- Brush the sides of the pasties with the egg (to create a seared shading during cooking).
- Put the pasties in the pre-warmed stove on a greased pan for 55 minutes.

LASAGNA

Lasagna, for the most part, contains two high-potassium foods (tomatoes and milk), making it a bad dish for those who need to follow a low-potassium diet. In this recipe we have used soya milk, which creates a similarly delectable white sauce yet is lower in potassium than cow's milk. You may also wish to top your lasagna with some ground mozzarella cheese, which is a lower-phosphate alternative to cheddar.

Ingredients:

- 1 tablespoon of vegetable or olive oil
- 250 grams (9 ounces) mince
- 1 onion, diced
- 3 carrots, ground
- 75 grams (2½ ounces) margarine or low-fat spread
- 75 grams (2½ ounces) plain flour
- 1 teaspoon English mustard
- 750 milliliters soya milk
- 2 garlic cloves, crushed
- 1 400-gram (14-ounce) tin of sliced tomatoes

- 1 low-salt bouillon cube (beef or vegetable)
- 100 milliliters water
- 250 grams (9 ounces) lasagna sheets
- 1 teaspoon oregano or basil (optional)
- Pepper
- 1 large bunch of ground mozzarella (optional)

Preparation:

- Preheat the broiler to 200°C (180°C Fan)/400°F.
- Heat a large griddle over medium heat and add the olive oil or vegetable oil. When hot, add the mince alongside a decent amount of pepper. Darken the mince for 5-6 minutes. Remove the mince from the skillet and set to the side.
- Add the onion and carrot to the griddle. Cook for 10 minutes.
- Liquify the margarine or spread in a pot over medium heat. When liquified, add the flour and mustard, then mix to blend well. Leave to cook over medium heat for 2 minutes, or until the blend becomes sticky.
- Pour the soya milk gradually into the pot to make a smooth white sauce. When all the soya milk is included, season with a bit of black pepper. Turn down the heat and leave to stew gently for 7 minutes.

- When the onions and carrots are softened, add the garlic to the skillet and cook for 2 minutes. Return the meat (in addition to any juices) to the dish and add the tomatoes, stock, and water. Combine everything, cover with a lid, and stew the sauce for 10 minutes until thickened slightly.
- To create the lasagna, place ¼ of the tomato sauce into the base of a small/medium-size heating dish. Top with a layer of lasagna sheets. Also, spoon another ¼ of the tomato sauce and top with 1/3 of the white sauce. Do this twice more, ending at the top with the last layer of white sauce.
- Cover with ground mozzarella, if you wish.
- Place into the preheated stove and cook for 30 minutes or until bubbling and the top darkens.

CABIN PIE

Those of you on a potassium restriction might be worried about the fact that this dish contains potato, a high-potassium food. However, we have lowered the amount of potato used for this recipe and replaced it with swede, a low-potassium food.

Ingredients:

- 400 grams (14 ounces) potatoes, for example, King Edward or Maris Piper, peeled and cut into pieces
- 400 grams (14 ounces) swede, peeled and cut into little pieces
- Margarine or low-fat olive oil spread
- Splash of milk
- Freshly ground black pepper
- 1 tablespoon vegetable or olive oil
- 1 onion, peeled, finely cleaved
- 1 garlic clove, peeled, squashed to a glue with the edge of a blade
- 1 large carrot, peeled, finely chopped
- 1 can of peas in water
- 2 teaspoons cleaved fresh thyme leaves
- 250-300 grams (9-11 ounces) mince
- 200 milliliters low-salt beef or vegetable stock
- 1 tablespoon tomato purée
- Freshly ground black pepper

Preparation:

- Preheat the broiler to 190°C (170°C Fan)/375°F.
- For the garnish, place the potatoes and swede into a large skillet of water. Bring to a boil and cook for 15-20 minutes, or until soft. When cooked, remove all of the water to eliminate the potassium.
- Add the spread to the cooked potato and swede and crush using a potato masher or ricer. Add the milk, a little at a time, and keep mashing until smooth. Season with freshly ground black pepper to taste. Put in a safe spot.
- Heat the oil in a large container over low to medium heat (for filling). Add the onion and fry for 8-10 minutes, or until softened.
- Add the garlic and carrot and fry for another 4-5 minutes, or until softened.
- Add mince to the container and fry for another 2-3 minutes, mixing consistently.
- Add the tomato purée and the stock and mix well. Bring the blend to a stew and keep stewing for another 4-5 minutes or until the sauce has thickened. Add the canned peas and season, to taste, with black pepper.
- Spoon the filling blend into a large ovenproof dish. Spread the mashed potato and swede blend over the filling in a smooth, even layer.

- Move to the stove and cook for 18-20 minutes, or until the garnish is dark-colored and the filling is cooked through.

SPAGHETTI BOLOGNESE

Spaghetti Bolognese is a great comfort food. While those on a low-potassium diet might stay away from it because it includes tomato and mushroom, it is actually okay to eat because it is usually served with spaghetti, a low-potassium food.

Ingredients:

- 1 tablespoon vegetable or olive oil
- 200 grams (7 ounces) mince
- 1 onion, finely sliced
- 4 large mushrooms, cut
- 1 carrot, ground
- 1 400-gram (14-ounce) can of sliced tomatoes
- 230 milliliters low-salt beef or vegetable stock
- 2 tablespoons tomato purée
- ½ teaspoon Worcestershire sauce
- 1 teaspoon freshly ground black pepper
- 1 teaspoon dried basil (optional)
- 300 grams (10½ ounces) whole-grain spaghetti

Preparation:

- Heat the olive oil in a large pan over medium heat. Add the mince and the onion and fry for 5 minutes, mixing once in a while until the mince is done and the onions have softened.
- Add mushrooms and carrot. Cook for around one minute. Add the canned tomatoes, stock, tomato purée, Worcestershire sauce, freshly ground black pepper, and basil (if using). Mix well and bring to a boil. Lower the heat to stew for 15-20 minutes, until the sauce has thickened.
- Place the whole-grain spaghetti in a deep pan brimming with salted boiling water. Cook as indicated by the instructions, then drain.
- To serve, separate the cooked spaghetti between four dishes. Spoon equivalent portions of Bolognese sauce over each.

STEW CON CARNE

This recipe contains kidney beans, which are high in potassium. However, as this supper includes rice, which is a much lower potassium food than options like potatoes, it is fine to consume. If you would like, you can exclude the kidney beans and try something else, like sweet corn.

Ingredients:

- 1 tablespoon vegetable or olive oil
- 1 onion, diced
- 2 garlic cloves, chopped
- 250 grams (9 ounces) mince
- Pepper
- ½ – 1 teaspoon stew drops, to taste
- 1 400-gram (14-ounce) tin of chopped tomatoes
- 300 milliliters of low-salt meat or vegetable stock
- ½ teaspoon dried blended herbs
- ½ teaspoon smoked paprika (optional)
- 1 400-g (14-ounce) can of red kidney beans, drained and washed
- 200 grams (7 ounces) long-grain rice or basmati rice

Preparation:

- Heat a large pan over medium heat. Add the oil and, when hot, fry the onion for 5 minutes, or until delicate and translucent. Add the garlic and cook for 2 minutes.
- Add the mince alongside a decent amount of pepper. Blend well and cook for 5-6 minutes, or until the meat is completely cooked. Add the beans, tomatoes, stock, dried blended herbs, and smoked paprika (if using). Mix to blend well and bring to a stew.
- Pour in the drained kidney beans and stew gently for 30 minutes, or until the stew con carne is thickened and rich. Taste and modify the flavoring as necessary.
- Cook the rice as per the directions on the box.

CONCLUSION

Eating well is a significant aspect of your treatment and can help you feel much better. In addition, a renal diet will allow you to avoid the inconveniences of your kidney disease, for example, excessive liquid, high blood potassium, bone disease, and weight loss. Because each individual is different and their needs are one-of-a-kind, the dietary suggestions in this book should be pursued only after you talk with your renal dietician. As stated before, kidney capacity is fundamental for expelling the waste material from the food that you eat. The kidneys discharge a dietary protein called urea, as well as sodium, potassium, and phosphate. These substances can develop in the body if kidney capacity is impeded. Following an exact diet can reduce this buildup.

Following a renal diet might seem to be overwhelming and somewhat prohibitive now and again. However, working with your doctor and a renal dietitian can help you create a renal diet exactly for your individual needs.